Nutrition For

HIV and Aging

Health and Immunity at 50+

Charlie Smigelski, RD
2013

©2013 Charlie Smigelski RD

ISBN-13:
978-1494471743

ISBN-10:
1494471744

Arlington, MA

Contents

Introduction	5
What Is Aging	5
The Stresses of HIV As A Chronic Infection	7
A Brief Lesson In Immune System Components	8
The Innate Immune System	8
The Acquired Immune System	9
The Glutathione Enzyme: Your Best Friend	11
Is It The Virus, The Meds, Or Aging; Could It Be Nutrition	13
The Foods To Keep You At you Best	13
Assembling A Really Good Diet For Yourself	15
Protein, to build a better body and brain	16
Vegetables restock your cells with minerals	18
Gettin' down with fruit	20
Foods for energy: starches and fats	22
Fuel for your brain and muscles: carbohydrates	23
You need to know the fats of life!	25
The Right Amount Of Food: understanding fuel needs	29
Physical Activity Raises Energy Needs	30
How much protein you will need each day	32
Protein Content of Common Foods	33
A food plan for someone who is 120 – 130 lbs.: ~1800 calories	35
A food plan for someone who is 150 – 165 lbs.: ~2300 calories	36
A food plan for someone who is 190 – 200 lbs.: ~2800 calories.	37
Designer Whey Protein Smoothies For Breakfast	38
Savory Vegetable Soup For Breakfast	38
Tell Me About Nutrition Supplements	39
Something about B-vitamins	39
The Case For Magnesium	40
The More Vitamin D The Better	41
Fur, Feathers, Cysteine and Glutathione	42
Some Insight Into The Negative News About Vitamin E	43
What would an incredibly nourishing diet look like?	45
Your decision to take vitamins rests on several ideas.	46
Should you take a multivitamin? I say, "Yes"	47
Nutrition Can Impact Rate of Aging	49
Medical Nutrition Therapy for Various Clinical Situations	50
Feed Your Head: Brain Cell Support	51
Brain Cell Plasticity	51
Fish Oils and Brain Cell Health	52
Cholesterol and Vascular Disease	57

Some Cholesterol Controversy	59
The Lyon Heart Study	61
The Details Of Heart Disease Risk in HIV Care	63
More Attention To Vitamin E	66
Low HDL is its own medical concern	67
Therapy With Essential Fatty Acids	68
Benefits Of Omega 3 EPA/DHA You Want To Be Aware Of	70
Omega 6 -- GLA fat benefits do not get enough medical attention	71
Every Possible Nutrition Step To Lower Cholesterol	72
Managing High Triglycerides	79
New Information: An Extra Heart Disease Risk Found In HIV Infection	82
Hypertension	83
The K+ Factor Diet	83
Heart Failure	87
Compound Nutritional Support For Impaired Hearts	89
Coenzyme Q10 in clinical cardiology: a long-term study.	91
Intestinal Health	92
Build A Better Bowel Movement	95
Help With Acid Reflux and GERD	95
Gut Rehab - Gut Ecology to Reduce Reflux	97
The Gut And On-going Immune Activation in HIV	99
The Gut Ecosystem and Better T Cell Counts	101
Bone Health, Osteoporosis, Risk of Fractures.	102
The Key Elements For Preventing Fractured Bones	103
Elevated Blood Sugar, Pre-diabetes and Diabetes	106
Nutrition and Metabolic Systems	106
Carbohydrate / sugar processing; Insulin Resistance And Diabetes	108
The Conditions That Generate Diabetes That Are Alterable Are:	111
Nutrients That Are Crucial To Insulin Working Well	113
Reversing Diabetic Complications	118
Being trapped in too many Diabetes Medicines	119
Food And Supplements That Support Liver Repair	124
Lipodystrophy Is Still Happening	125
Keeping Mitochondria In Good Condition	127
Your Lipodystrophy Treatment Roadmap (as of 2013)	130
Tiredness and fatigue remedy	130
Reducing Neuropathy	131
Energy Healing With Tong Ren Therapy	133
Brainwave Entrainment For Synchronicity.	134
Conclusion	134
Appendix 1 All Possible Supplements	136
Appendix 2 Practical Supplement Intervention	137
Appendix 3 Guide To Groceries	138

Introduction

Is It Aging ... Is It HIV ... Is It The Meds ... ? Yes, Yes, & Yes.

All too often, caring for oneself when HIV-positive, seems like moving through a rugged, uncharted wilderness. Most people are feeling a little more relaxed about managing the virus these days. However, the ability to coast along comfortably never seems to last as long as would be nice. Whenever some new health glitch arises: high blood pressure, acid reflux, more fatigue, it can feel like a setback. The thought arises, "Uh oh, will this be just a small issue to handle, or will it be another chronic issue to contend with?"

Meanwhile, there are some gloomy statistics out there. Rates of coronary artery disease development, and of cognitive decline are higher in people with HIV infection. This is especially true for those who have been positive for a number of years and are now over age 50. Conditions like asthma, high cholesterol, and hypertension sometimes seem harder to manage, too. When something new comes along, both clinicians and consumers are wondering, "Is it ageing; is it HIV?" The answer is, "It's likely both." You can't change either of those conditions, but at this stage of the game, nutritional solutions may be the most important intervention in problem solving new or festering medical conditions. It is certainly the least toxic, and usually the cheapest. The rest of the story is that for everyone, positive or not, age 50 is kind of a nutrition and aging threshold. Many body systems start to "act" older at this age. The liver and kidneys just aren't acting as energetic as they once could. Add on the extra demands of a busy immune system and the picture is more complex. As you read on, hopefully you will see how nutrition may be the solution to many glitches you've been experiencing, and possibly getting frustrated with.

What Is Aging?

What causes ageing is still a subject of debate. Meanwhile, several of the major concepts of aging do relate to events in HIV infection. Accumulated damage from free radicals and singlet oxygen species seems to be one likely aging mechanism.[1] What does this mean? Here is a simple explanation. Sunlight is energy. That energy is captured in plants, becoming the electrons in the atoms and molecules of our food. We digest the food, and the energy is released, but sometimes a few of the electrons spin out of orbit and cause damage. The damage is 'oxidative stress'; the out of control particles are 'free radicals'. An analogy: rust is the damage happening when stray electrons hit metals. We have some metals in us that rust. The stray electrons also cause us to brown, like the ends of a roast beef. The caramelization in us is charmingly called A.G.E.-- advanced glycation endproducts. Another mechanism of aging is changes in gene structures and in genetic expression.[2] A combination of the two is also possible. Stray electrons can cause damage in more than one bit of cell structure.[3] A new focus in aging is mitochondrial malfunction; the cumulative stray electron damage has particular bearing on these parts of cells.[4]

Mitochondria are the structures within cells where food energy (electrons) are transformed to ATP, the body's energy currency for nerves and muscles. Messed up mitochondria means slower energy production, which has consequences for cells all over the body. One other concept in aging is impaired glutathione activity, leading to a pro-oxidant state in cells.[5] Glutathione (GSH) is the major anti-oxidant enzyme in eyeballs, lungs, liver, kidneys, and in the blood stream. In aging it seems the body is not able to generate GSH as fast as it once could. This means that in times of stressed metabolisms, like when something is generating a lot of stray electrons (free radicals), the system can't keep up, and more rust/corrosion happens. So this is the "science" of aging, but what about the practical implications?

As people accumulate more years of life, they realize that their bodies do not respond to tasks and stresses as well as they used to. They can't jog up a flight of stairs the way they used to; they seem to take longer to heal from bruises, cuts, and colds. People simply declare these events the result of aging. Technically, a number of physiological processes change as people age. Fundamental is that protein synthesis is slowed as we age. Genetic blueprints are not read with as much precision as when we were young.[6] Cells also don't reproduce as exactly as they once did. Body parts will work a little less well, like lungs become less elastic, so a deep breath doesn't deliver as much oxygen as it used to.[7] Kidney filtration rate slows, meaning some drugs are slower to process.[8] Gut flora, (intestinal good bacteria) population may also change, leading to a set of species that are less prone to reducing inflammation.[9] (On page 95, you can read the good news: supplementation with probiotics--beneficial gut bacteria pills--can reverse the problem.)[10] As you would expect, the corrosive effect of years of stray electrons takes its toll on arteries. Cholesterol deposits in the scratched up lining of blood vessels leads to "hardening of the arteries" and diminished flow of blood.[11] This is the basis of heart disease. Subtle corrosions, happening all over the body, are causing what people sense as older age.

Relevant to HIV, the slower protein assembly events impact immune cells, causing what is called "immune senescence" (immune aging).[12] The science of really understanding immune system components is young and evolving. We do know that aging plays out, first, as inability to activate naïve T cells and generate memory T cells.[13] CD4 T cells are the "generals" that direct activities of the acquired immune system. The "soldiers" doing battle against virus are CD8 cells. Again with age, the ability of CD8 cells to multiply diminishes. In technical words: there is a "CD8+ T-cell replicative senescence in human aging."[14] A consequence of this is a lapse into a more pro-inflammatory state in aging.[15] Many cells have a genetically determined number of reproductions they are capable of. Telomeres are the part of the genes that code for this reproductive capacity. If you are interested in how the immune system works, what is happening with telomeres and CD cell populations in ageing in general makes for fascinating reading. What is also nice to see is that people are looking at telomeres in HIV infection. Researchers are observing that HIV-specific CD8 cell telomeres are shortening, again this means aging.[16] What is relevant to this book is that good nutrition impacts telomere length in beneficial way.[17] Nutrients can modulate oxidative stress and inflammation, which are the forces that adversely affect all parts of DNA, including telomeres. What is also exciting is that people are working on sophisticated dietary supplements that can slow aging and positively impact immune cell behaviors.[18] The science is showing that what we expect to be deterioration of immune capability with age can be modified. When older people are newly diagnosed with HIV, their immune recovery is known to be slower than what occurs in younger people.[19] The good news is that anti-HIV medicines still do work in older people. The even better news is that smart nutritional support can be significantly effective here too.

The Stresses of HIV As A Chronic Infection

Chronic infection in general seems to speed up the ageing process. HIV disease is no exception. For many people, viral loads are undetectable, and CD4 T cell counts are in the healthy range. For others, drug-resistant virus and not sufficiently powerful meds are leaving people with detectable virus, and sub-optimal T cell counts. In both sets of people, other glitches in the system are appearing.[20] Those glitches can be body fat loss, intestinal problems, or debilitating fatigue.[21] One of the HIV infection events very much on peoples' minds is the apparent accelerated rate of brain senescence. Brain volume is connected to brain function and mental competence. Both age and HIV cause shrinking of various brain parts.[22] Shrinking of both white and gray matter seems to be happening at an earlier age in people with HIV, compared to people who are HIV negative.[23] Again, this is a condition where good nutrition can have a beneficial effect.

Finally, while the accelerated risk of atherosclerosis (narrowing of blood vessels) seems like a new focus, initial reports date back over a decade.[24] Traditional risk factors for vascular problems, like cigarette smoking, plus higher cholesterol and lower HDL, are still are strong predictors of coronary artery disease (CAD). At the same time, a 2010 Italian study noted that HIV infection itself seems to age people an extra 7.6 years prior to their going on HAART therapy.[25] This study also noted that waist circumference was tied to risk of arterial disease. This will be a topic of discussion in upcoming chapters. A little publicized mechanism of atherosclerosis in HIV infection is how the protease inhibitors provoke CD36 (foam) cell activity, leading to more laying down of cholesterol plaque.[26] This sclerosing process is totally separate from the effect that elevated lipids like high cholesterol may have on arterial disease. Later on, read about how vitamin E supplements can stop the unwanted CD36 cell activity. The nutritional agenda, still, involves improving repair capacity whenever possible, to either prevent or slow the damaging process.

Metabolic Events to Appreciate in HIV and Aging

Free radicals generated by a busy immune system are the issue to keep in mind. While T Cell numbers can be good, and viral load undectable, there is still some on-going immune activity, meaning extra stray electrons are zooming around. Here are the basics of the ongoing anti-viral fight the body is waging.

A Brief Lesson in Immune System Components

The Innate Immune System

There are several layers to the immune system. It is the "innate immune system" that first confronts invading viruses like HIV, Hep C, a cold or the flu. The prime players here are the Natural Killer (NK) cells of the Innate Immune System. These are cells that are roving through the body at all times, and ready to fight all kinds of bad cells: germs, viruses, bacteria, fledgling cancer cells. They don't multiply too quickly, and are somewhat crude in their killing capacity; their talent is that they are agile, and can confront anything. Just a few years ago, some Boston researchers reported important new insights into NK cell activity. I want to quote them,

> "Increasing evidence supports the notion that the innate immune response, and in particular, natural killer cells, play a central role in determining the quality of the host immune response to infection. In this review we highlight recent evidence that suggests that NK cells influence the clinical fate of HIV-infected individuals."[27]

What happens to NK cells as people age is not totally clear, but the trend is to get more sluggish and less numerous.[28] The question is whether this decline is inevitable, or a function of nutritional deficiency? Meanwhile NK cells also make chemical signals – cytokines – that will start up the activities of the Acquired Immune System. Just so you know, cytokines have names like Interleukin 1, Interleukin 2, Interleukin 6, Interferon, and Tumor Necrosis Factor alpha. The abbreviations are: IL_1, IL_2, Il_6, IFN, and TNFa. These cytokines tell the body to produce certain kinds of immune cells. They also tell the body how to fuel the immune cells, so you should appreciate that they have an effect on fat cell inventory and sugar metabolism. Cytokines have quite a dynamic effect on the body. The ache you feel when you have the flu comes for the IL_2 response to the invading virus. You may already know that IFN injections that people get as part of Hepatitis treatment also cause ache, fatigue and depression. Back to the story here: NK cells release cytokines that tell the body to make T cells.

The Acquired Immune System

The acquired immune system is also known as the "adaptive" immune system. This means the body makes cells that are specially crafted to defeat whatever the germ invader is. NK cells, as mentioned above, are good generalists, but having specialists around makes for an even more robust immune response. As you see in the diagram below, T cells start out in a Th0, blank slate form. In HIV infection, the cytokine chemical signals arriving from NK and a few other cells, will direct the T cells to a Th1 response. This means making CD4 T cells and also CD8 T cells, [also called Cytotoxic T Lymphocytes (CTL's)]. Think of CD4 T cells as the generals that direct the immune response, and CD8 cells as the soldiers doing the work of fighting virus.

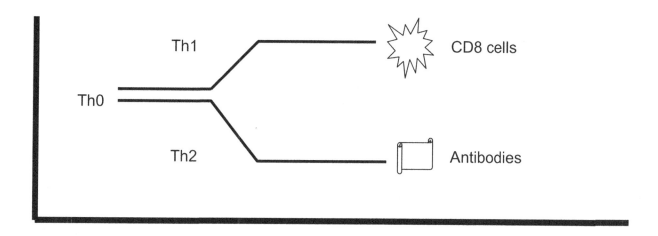

The Th1 and Th2 Aspects Of The Acquired Immune Response

When the Th1 system doesn't totally conquer the invading germs, or sometimes just to bat clean up, the Th2 system comes into play, making antibodies. An example, we conquer measles with Th1 response, but the Th2 antibodies keeps measles squelched. Antibodies are also called "immune globulins". You might have heard that people get "gamma globulin" shots when exposed to Hepatitis B, to help them recover from the infection faster. Globulins come in various forms, and get letter titles: IgA, IgE, IgG are some examples.

A smaller part of the body's anti-HIV (and anti-Hep C) immune activity is the Th2 response, making antibodies to these viruses. Think of antibodies as custom clamps that grab a virus and render it impotent. The problem is, these two viruses can keep changing their outward coats, so the custom antibodies no longer match up to the viruses' coatings, and the virus keeps escaping control. **The continuous creation and deterioration of ineffective antibody cells is a major source of the chronic inflammation seen in HIV infection.**[29] Deterioration of these antibodies is a continuous sourse of free radicals, i.e. stray electrons.

As you would imagine, the immune system is sensitive to nutrition status of the body. The Th1 response relies on adequate amounts of zinc, selenium, and glutathione, a major antioxidant enzyme. [Glutathione levels are dependant on adequate protein and certain amino acids, plus vitamin C and vitamin E in the diet.] An important nutritional concept is that if the Th1 cell system runs low in zinc, selenium or glutathione, there is a shift to the Th2 response. Another important concept here, first described in a 1996 article: over time, there is an observed shift from Th1 to Th2 response in HIV infection. These authors point out that a balance of both Th1 and Th2 responses is more likely to keep the immune response functioning better.[30] No one knows whether the observed shift away from the Th1 to Th2 is something that HIV itself causes, or whether it is just the Th1 system running out of nutrients.

Adding a selenium molecule to the antioxidant Glutathine enzyme produces a more specialized antioxidant called Glutathione peroxidase, abbreviated GSX. Lower glutathione levels were connected to impaired survival in the pre-HAART era.[31] Stimulation of intestinal glutathione peroxide can lower Hep C viral load.[32] Lower levels of GPX are also connected to higher HIV viral load, and some researchers suggest nutritional support of GSX could be an element of anti-viral therapy.[33]

The immune response to HIV infection remains so complex. There are a small number of people who have never needed anti-HIV meds, despite years of infection. These people are "elite controllers". They have Th2 antibodies that successfully manage to squelch the virus. Duplicating those antibodies has so far eluded scientists; this is one reason why a vaccine has not yet happened yet. Meanwhile, for the rest of people living with HIV, again, it is a blend of NK cells and Th1-generated CD8 cells that combats the virus. In this case, a lapse to more Th2 activity has negative consequences. People who shift to the more Th2 response cytokine message seem to make more CCR5 surface marker T cells, making it easier for HIV to enter CD4 cells, and cause more rapid progression in disease.[34] Luckily, researchers are experimenting with compounds that either block excessive Th2 action,[35] or nurture stronger Th1 activity. The supportive compounds include nutritional materials, like N-acetylcysteine (NAC), which is the limiting amino acid in production of glutathione.[36]

Here is one quick point of nutritional interest. The immune system is working harder when more Th2 cytokines are present. People feel sicker: like the body aches of the flu. The Th2 response is directed by the cytokines (chemical messengers) Interleukin 4, Interleukin 5 and Interleukin 6. These cytokines cause more damage to muscles and the liver, as they are directing a flood of antibodies into an infected area. For example, there is more Interleukin 6 present in cirrhosis of the liver from hepatitis B. Crohn's disease, multiple sclerosis and rheumatoid arthritis "flare ups" are associated with more Il_6 of the Th2 response. [The nutritional strategy to prevent flare-ups is to keep the Th1 response system well-nourished, so there is less risk of a lapse into the more stressful Th2 activity. You also see more Th2 cytokine activity in HIV lipodystrophy.

I will discuss food and supplement vitamins for the best Th1 immune activity in future pages. I want to point out a few facts here, though. Remember, Th1 action depends on a healthy intake of selenium, zinc and antioxidants like vit C and vit E. After oysters, beef is the best source of zinc in the diet. Not many people are routinely eating oysters, and the public health message is to eat less beef. As a result, zinc intake in America is low for many people. The RDA is 12 mg for women, and 15 mg for men. Half (50%) of America eats 10 mg a day or less! Fish is the best source of selenium, and again, 50% of Americans eat no fish. A New Jersey study back in 1996 reported 20% of the HIV+ people they researched had low blood levels of vitamin C.[37] Taking some vitamin supplements to cover these common deficits is a great idea. See page 46 to get an idea of what might be best for you.

Echinacea and other immune boosting agents.

Boosting the immune system with other supplements often sounds like a great idea in advertisements. It is not. People think of Echinacea and other items as good for the immune system. Excess immune system stimulation can be counterproductive. We know that too much TNFa is associated with higher risk of anti-HIV drug treatment failure.[38] We know excess TNFa is a part of lipodystrophy. You want the immune system simply competent, not overactive. You fuel the Th1 response, so that it is quick, efficient and accurate, and not excessively busy. You don't want additional immune activation that would summon Th2 activity. Think of this analogy. When your room is cold, you may turn up the thermostat to make the furnace run. If there is no oil in the tank, no matter how much you spin the dial on the thermostat, the furnace won't fire up. In HIV and Hep C care, there is already plenty of immune stimulation i.e. thermostat ON switch activity; the issue is more likely not enough nutrients (fuel) to support immune cells. In general, do not spend money on immune stimulating agents. Later on, you'll read about the amino acid L-glutamine as a supplement. This is fuel for immune cells. It also improves Interleukin 2 receptor function. People see this as "immune boosting" but its true action is that it's energy for cells that may be running low on fuel.[39]

The Glutathione Enzyme ... get to know your (new) best friend

Become comfortable with the word Glutathione, abbreviated GSH. The Glutathione enzyme is crucial to many body systems. An enzyme is a protein compound that is essentially a piece of working equipment that helps chemical reactions happen. It processes things. Example: a digestive enzyme called "lipase" breaks down the fat molecules in food to small particles so they can be absorbed through the gut wall. The launching of both CD4 and CS8 cells for the Th1 response depends on adequate supply of GSH.[40] The cytotoxicity (killing capacity) of both T cells and Natural Killer (NK) cells depends on having adequate amounts of GSH, too.[41] GSH is the major antioxidant enzyme that is taming stray electrons in lungs,[42] liver, and kidneys; it keeps eyes protected from free radical damage too.[43] As mentioned before, with a selenium molecule attached, it becomes glutathione peroxidase--GSX: another important antioxidant compound.[44]

Glutathione levels are low in HIV-infected people,[45] as well as in those with HCV, (Hepatitis C).[46] The effect is compounded in co-infected people.[47] Running low in glutathione precedes elevations in ALT and hepatic ferritin (iron) accumulation in people with HCV.[48] (Iron in the liver is likely to rust from stray electrons, and cause scarring and raise cancer risk.) Remember, having higher gut glutathione peroxidase levels and better general antioxidant levels keeps HCV viral load lower.[49] While it seems that Hep C viral load is not correlated with rate or degree of liver cell damage and cirrhosis risk, elevation in liver enzymes, like ALT, does increase risk of liver (hepatocellular) cancer.[50][51][52] As you would expect, a busy immune system consumes more nutrients, so there are vitamin deficits, which can leave liver cells open to more damage from toxic materials.[53] Once again, this is a place where smart nutritional care can yield positive results. More info on glutathione support is yet to come. Here in the case for liver, actually keeping iron-intake low to the point of near anemia can seriously reduce liver cancer risk for people with cirrhosis.[54] I want you to know, glutathione status is hugely important to anyone worried about liver health and improving T cell count.

Glutathione status is not part of common health evaluations the way cholesterol or C-Reactive Protein numbers are, but in the case of chronic infection, please do appreciate that if GSH levels become low, major immune and repair systems will struggle. It matters to so many body functions; especially ones that people feel are part of the accelerated aging of HIV infection. GSH is a part of insulin messaging, so relates to diabetes risk.[55] GSH status affects functional cardiac problems like atrial fibrillation.[56] There is even a role in eye health, like modulating the progression of macular degeneration.[57] Long-term infection means cumulative stray electron damage. Anti-HIV medicines also generate oxidative stress, leading to changes in the cells lining arteries that over time generate heart disease.[58] The bottom line is that protein synthesis is slowed in aging: this includes GSH synthesis. The good news is, that nutritional supplementation can reverse the problem.[59] I will discuss whey protein and N-acetylcysteine (NAC) for GSH support later on (page 42).

As you think about immune function, body repair capacity, and aging, you want to have some knowledge about when and how to support the antioxidant enzyme Glutathione.

Support For People With A Chronic Infection

Is It The Virus, Is It The Meds, Is It Aging; Could It Be Nutrition?

"HIV infection as a chronic manageable disease" is a common phrase now. Clearly this is good news, but it has an edge. You are living with the edge. The complication is, when things like diabetes, high blood pressure or bone loss happen, you get confused. Is this a result of the HIV infection itself, the anti-HIV meds, or the process of aging? The answer is likely yes, yes, and yes. Too often, medical providers don't understand the nutritional part of chronic infection and of simple aging. Both have a big malnutrition component. For the next chapters, I will discuss aging and nutrition, and add on the elements that relate to HIV and Comprehensive Anti-Retroviral Therapy: cART or HAART. The goal is that you will be better nourished; your whole body, and especially your immune and antioxidant systems will operate better. After reading this book, you can decipher whether some medical blip is an HIV or cART event, or an aging issue; and you'll have a nutritional solution in either case.

Introduction: The Food Part Of Nutrition To Keep You At you Best

The next section here is about food for repairing you. Last night's supper and evening snacks were supposed to restore your body while you slept. Maybe food is repairing legs from yesterday's "brisk walk" that your doctor has prescribed for you. So, how did you do? Are you feeling fit today? Maybe you're sluggish because the magnesium or B-vitamins weren't there at 4 am, when the protein assembly line needed a nutritional nudge to link some amino acids into key contractile muscle fibers? At the end of the workday, are your ankles a little puffy, fluid pooling there at the far end of your body, because your heart just doesn't have enough oomph to pump the liquids around this corner (at your feet), and back up your calves and thighs? It is the simple truth: the groceries you buy, the meals and snacks you eat, the vitamins you take; these are what keeps your muscle, bone, brain and immune cells operating at their best. Your nutrition choices, past and present, decide the performance quality of your cells, and after age 50, they matter even more.

Your doctor often suggests medicines when you have complaints. You take a pill to stop the pain of arthritis. The drug stops the hurt; but doesn't help the underlying problem: failure of the joint cells to repair. Remember, you are not suffering from an ibuprofen deficiency; you have an "itis," an inflammation, because cells are not mending well enough. As many of you know, the drugs have their own set of complications, usually some undesirable side effects. At this point in life, you want to focus on having all systems at their metabolic optimum; otherwise the stack of pills for managing symptoms keeps mounting. The food section coming up details the foods you could eat, for best repair. In a later section, I discuss the vitamins and other supplements you can take to repair you as well as possible.

This section is about smart food and nutrition choices. Don't let the advice lapse into feeling like yet another set of food rules to live by. View it, instead, as ideas to move you into a stronger place. Food is still supposed to be fun. It can have tremendous spiritual and psychological power too. It's the cornerstone of Maslow's *Hierarchy of Needs*.[60] We're pretty grumpy characters if we're deprived of food for many hours or days. Food brightens our mood too: succulent strawberries and luscious whip cream on a crispy sweet biscuit perk up a summer supper, for sure. OK, eat up.

Here is a core idea, a fundamental concept to utilize in making most of your food choices. Have what you eat be food that your caveman/cavewoman genes are expecting to receive, to do the work of replenishing your system today. We carry the gene product of about 100,000 years of evolution as homosapiens.[61]

For your body to function at its best, have the food you eat supply the materials that your caveman/cavewoman genes are expecting.

There is also the opposite concept: when thinking about what to eat, ask yourself whether this food will hassle your body, and be more of a burden on repair systems? The idea is not to make a health food freak of you, but a lot of what passes for routine cuisine these days is either lacking in key repair nutrients, or providing annoying (meaning mildly toxic) stuff for the body.

Will the food you are about to eat hinder the repair systems or be a burden to the operating cells of your body?

Keep Food Enjoyable

One more perspective: let's be practical and realistic, but also emotional and spiritual. As you pull breakfast or lunch together, what are you really nourishing? There is the physical part of you that may be about to go out and pedal a bicycle for an hour or two, or go sit through a ninety-minute committee meeting. Both activities require steady fuel and energy." A smart blend of fats, carbohydrates and protein will get you there.

To stay focused on eating well for the long haul, you'd do well to also have another mental component to your food selection process. Do you actually look forward to breakfast, or lunch? Why, or why not? Could you see food as fun: the tropical smell of mango, the summer sweet of blueberries, to start your day off on a good note? Will it be yet another turkey sandwich for lunch today, on whole wheat, lettuce,

Have the food you eat be nourishing to your cells, as well as to the psychological and spiritual you.

tomato, and mustard ... same as the last 17 weeks? If lunch were a little more fun and exciting, what would that do for your well being today? Would a salad of black beans, corn, diced tomato and maple-smoked chicken sausage, arranged on baby spinach leaves with cilantro, feel just a little more fun? Is it that much extra work to make the salad at home and bring it to the office, or would just some planning ahead make it happen? Maybe you start with gourmet Thursdays, just to perk up the latter part of the workweek? This meal can nourish your arms and legs, but also feed the happy section in your brain cells for the next few hours.

A Guide to Groceries and Eating:

[handwritten note: mention this in bigger/broader points]

The next dozen or so pages of this book discuss food groups and individual items within those categories. Read them so you can learn about particularly good elements in certain choices, so you might find foods you already like, and that are actually especially good for you.

Then will come some pages with sample menus for the day. Some recipes will be sprinkled though the pages, so you can enjoy some new foods in a tasty way.

Assembling a really good diet for yourself

As you think about eating well, assemble your daily diet in a series of steps.

1. Figure out **proteins**, and have them at all three meals: breakfast, lunch, and dinner. These are foods for structure. As we age, research is showing that we need more protein, not less.[62] No breakfast, then have the protein at an evening snack.

2. Plan on eating a lot of **vegetables** at both lunch and dinner; you need more vegetables than you think, and you likely can't meet all your needs having them just at supper. [63] [64]

3. Stock up on **fruits.** You want to eat them 3-4 times a day. Remember 7 days a week, times 3 per day is a lot: 21 fruit items in your grocery cart this week.

4. Nuts and seeds have a lot of calories, but they also contain essential oils that form cell membranes and brain insulation. A good idea is eating one handful of **nuts** and one of **seeds** every day.

5. Pick **starches** (carbohydrates) as the remaining part of your fuel needs. Select wisely; you need the carbs for fuel, but think about portions. In aging, over-sized servings of starches tend to turn to fat faster.[65]

More details on assembling a food plan come on pages 35 to 37.

essential! ↓

Protein, to build a better body and brain

[Your body is in a constant state of renewal.] You are making new liver, intestine and skin cells every day. You are also making millions of immune cells to fight off the virus, plus the colds or other germs you get from living in the modern world. Also, you are repairing muscle and bone cells. All these body parts require protein for repair. Protein needs rise as we age. Loss of muscle, known as «sarcopenia» is a much bigger problem than people and doctors appreciate [66] In a Connecticut study, 20% people over 64 showed signifcant muscle loss, and over age 80, the numbers were 30% and higher. In normal aging, bone loss, osteoporosis, gets a lot of publicity because pharmaceutical companies have increased direct to consumer advertizing budgets to promote bone growth drugs,[67] but subtle loss of muscle is a far more important clinical issue. [Bone loss in HIV is about the meds, and about protein too.]

Your body is expecting you to crawl out of your hut or cave this morning, go over to the river, lake or ocean, smack a fish over the head, or grab some clams, and start dining. Maybe you'll sneak up on a bird, grab it and eat it. One important concept here: having protein for breakfast is a critical part of your good nutrition plan. Whey protein is a handy and healthy choice. At any meal, fish and seafood are always good protein. Fish with omega 3 oils is extra good. Bird is pretty good too. Just so you know, tuna does not have much omega 3. Have wild Alaskan salmon instead. See recipe on page 35. You may have been told that shrimp or other shellfish have a lot of cholesterol, so avoid them: not true. These contain plant sterols, but not excessive cholesterol. Cook them in a low fat way, and enjoy. Shrimp with cocktail sauce: perfect. Scallops seared in a pan with a little olive oil and garlic: excellent.

The way to think about choosing proteins, (and many other good foods), is to think back to selections that reflect caveman era choices.

There are modern animals, like cows and sheep that we eat, but these now have more saturated fat than the body is accustomed to dealing with. In the olden days, people chased down deer or wild boar, but the flesh was very lean when they grew in their natural state. They were grass-fed, meaning they contain omega 3 fats! Cheese is another whole story. In the famous Mediterranean Diet, in its purest form on the island of Crete, even the cheese and ice cream have omega 3 fats, because all the dairy producing animals were grass fed. Their dairy tends to come from goat and sheep milk, as another point of interest.[68] Back here in the US, the saturated fat from dairy is not so benign. Stick to lower fat dairy items when you can, and see full fat cheese as an occasional treat. If eating beef or lamb, whenever you can, buy «grass-fed» and free of antibiotics. It is leaner, and has omega 3 fats: so no worries.

Remember the simple idea: your body expects much of your protein to come from ocean, or streams and rivers. Proteins with saturated fat change the physical and metabolic performance of your cells. Don't add the hassel of coping with that thick grease to the work of repairing you. Keep the added burden to a few events per week.

Protein concepts

When you think about eating to repair your body, you want to think about eating proteins from the streams, lakes and oceans, or low fat land items.

The more you eat from the upper part of the list at right, the better off you are.

The fish at the top of the list have more "omega-3 oils, which have natural anti-inflammatory properties. Other fish are still great choices, because they are low fat and have minimal saturated fat. Seafood is lean as well. Enjoy shrimp and scallops. Their cholesterol content is not an issue, as was once thought.

You want to eat protein at breakfast, lunch, and dinner.

Designer whey protein is a great repair protein. Blend it with fruit for smoothies at breakfast.

Salmon
Sardines
Herring
Mackerel
Trout

Cod
Haddock
Shrimp
Scallops
Lobster
Clams
Mussels
(Tuna)

Whey protein powder
Egg whites
Low fat cottage cheese
Lite cheeses
Soy powder or Tofu
Soy burgers

Turkey breast
Turkey ham
Turkey sausage
Chicken breast
Chicken legs
Chicken thighs
Pork tenderloin
Pork chops
Omega 3 eggs

Lamb chops
Lean hamburger
Round steak
Filet mignon
Sirloin steak

Vegetables restock your cells with minerals

Back to the caveman idea: in the old days, people got huge amounts of nutrition in vegetables. They wandered around munching leaves and shoots like Swiss chard, collards, and asparagus all day. Imagine eating 5 or 6 bags of leaves, I mean salad, in a day. You probably won't do this now, but it is what your body is somewhat expecting, is certainly ready for, and likes to get. You often hear about «The Mediterranean Diet» based on the food intake of people on the island of Crete. Well, people there seem to consume 245 kilograms of vegetables per year, compared to the 150 in Italy and France, and 90 in Finland.[69] Do some math: 2.2 lbs X 245 kg = ~ 540 lbs ! divided by 365 ... 1.5 lbs per day ! So, don't be patttting yourself on the back because you ate a splash of lettuce and tomato on your sandwich. When you have 2 quarts of salad, or 3 huge carrots, or 2 tomatoes and a whole green pepper at lunch, then you get to feel proud. I'll say it again, «Eat a serious amount of veges daily.»

Eating many minerals, like potassium, magnesium, selenium and copper is the key to ideal operation of all kinds of hormones and repair enzymes. Blood pressure stays lower, insulin manages blood sugar better, and bones rebuild better, all thanks to the crucial amounts of minerals in vegetables.

There is always room to be doing better with eating vegetables. The cafeteria at work may not have a great selection, but do what you can. If the vegetables are kind of soft and tired, toss them in some soup to make them taste a little better.

At the salad bar, what vegetables look good today? The lettuce looks limp, so maybe your salad is just celery and mushrooms: fine; those two foods are very good blood pressure therapy. Eat a cereal bowl size portion. Another day it may be just a salad of beets and chopped onion. This is still a useful nutritional move.

**Eat vegetables at both lunch and supper,
and even as part of a snack if you can.**

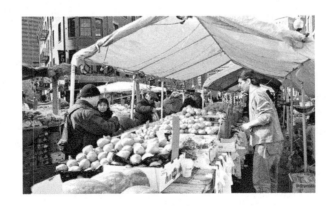

Here's the word on vegetables

Here is a list of vegetables to remind you of the many choices you have.

All vegetables give you some good nutrition, plus fiber.

In this list, the vegetables at the top are the ones with the most vitamins or minerals or both.

You might be someone who is just not into eating vegetables. At least try to have a small amount of something high on the list. Then eat an extra piece of fruit each day, to make up for the fiber you are missing.

While fresh and frozen are the best, even canned vegetables still offer some minerals and fiber. By the way, the gooey fiber in okra and eggplant is especially good for lowering cholesterol.

Eat at least a cup of vegetables at both lunch and supper. More as snacks is good, too.

Ever tried Swiss chard? It's a super-food: serious magnesium content.

Carrots
Broccoli
Spinach
Winter squash
Parsley
Kale
Swiss chard
Collard greens
Dandelion
   Greens
Purslane

Asparagus
Bok choy
Brussels
   sprouts
Cabbage
Cauliflower
Dark green
   Lettuce
Eggplant
Green/yellow beans
Green/red peppers
Mushrooms
Mustard greens
Okra
Pea pods
Tomatoes
Tomato sauce
Celery
Onion
Parsnip
Summer squash
Zucchini squash

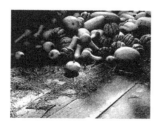

Gettin' down with fruit

Imagine being out wandering the countryside, coming across a clump of wild strawberries on a warm sunny day. Maybe as you pass a stream, you find a bush full of blueberries, perfect for snacking. You sit down and munch away. Fruit and berries must be a regular part of your snacking routine. Your body has processed this sugar for tens of thousands of years. In cave people times, there were no bagels, crackers, cookies and cupcakes to snack on. These are modern inventions; they are not particularly progress either.

If you are the boss and are looking for cheap fuel for the workers building a pyramid in Egypt, or a great wall in China, bread and rice do the trick. Grains have become popular in the past few thousand years, but food for poor laborers is not what makes you the healthiest, though. The point of the story is that fruit is the ideal fuel for snacks, it is rich in minerals and vitamins. You will still have grains in your diet, but this is just an argument for why you need to be snacking on fruits, multiple times a day, then adding grains after that.

Another concept: all the colors -- the pigments -- in fruit (and vegetables) have anti-oxidant properties. Eating more antioxidants translates into less stray electron damage. In his book *What Color Is Your Diet?* David Heber, MD, PhD. explains the idea more.[70] He's brilliant. Think red, orange, blue, green, yellow, brown foods.

Many people worry about how sweet bananas are, and whether they provoke too much insulin response. For people worried about blood sugar responses, eat solid fruits, don't drink juices. Also, don't eat fruits and starches/grains at the same meal or snack. Having 100 calorie servings, even of dried fruits, won't burden your blood sugar management system. Eat fruits with nuts, seeds or protein, to slow their digestion, and reduce the speed at which they raise your blood sugar.

[Just a side note, when muscles are all warmed up from physical exercise, they absorb blood sugars easier, and need less insulin to help process the sugar in the blood. Fruit snacks during walks and bike rides are perfect.]

Nuts and berries were a routine part of daily fuel for hunters and gatherers. People in the olden days ate at least 4 or 5 servings of fruit a day, and stayed healthy and got you here. You do the same, to stay in a good state of repair.

So many fruits, and lots of time!

Here is a list of fruits, to remind you of the many choices you have. Fresh, canned and dried all work.

Frozen berries, blended with Designer Whey protein, make excellent breakfast smoothies.

Behind the scenes, fruit keeps intestine cells in good shape, and keeps skin healthier. Eating fruit nurtures the beneficial bacteria living in the gut and all over the body.

You need to eat fruit at least 3 times a day, maybe more. The *fruits have more pectin, which lowers cholesterol too.

Juices are over-rated. They are missing the fiber and minerals of solid fruits. Many are made with apple and white grape juice concentrates: this means sugar-water.

Drink water or seltzer for thirst, and eat solid fruits for health.

Modest, 4oz., servings of juice are about all you can justify.

Oranges
Grapefruit
Bananas*

Apricots
Cantaloupe
Clementines
Mangos
Nectarines
Papaya
Peaches
Blueberries
Strawberries
Raspberries
Red grapes
Honeydew melon
Kiwis
Watermelon
Apples*
Pears*
Applesauce*
Pineapple

Dates
Figs
Raisins
Cran-raisins

Modest 4oz. servings:
  Orange juice
  Apricot nectar
  Pineapple juice
  Red grape juice
  Pomegranate juice

 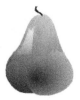

Foods for energy: *starches and fats*

You have read about protein to repair yourself. You have read about fruits and vegetables to support enzymes and hormones that keep your body healthy.

Now think about food for energy. The work of fueling your brain, your kidneys, your eyes, and you muscles comes mostly from starches and somewhat from fats.

Starches are foods like kidney beans, (sweet) potatoes, bread, noodles, pasta and rice. Starch, plus grease and sugar, equals muffins, cakes and cookies.

Fats come in nuts and seeds, and in oils. Fats are also found in spreads, like butter, margarine, and cream cheese. Fats also come from fried foods, like French fries, potato chips and corn chips. You probably remember that fats are already built into the fish, chicken, meats and cheese you eat too.

When it comes to how much to eat for the fuel foods, think about your activity level. The average person, not getting much exercise or physical activity, needs to take it easy in both the amount of fats and starch in his or her diet. If you are reading this book, hopefully you are someone who does a smart amout of physical fitness activity More information about fuel and exercise comes on pages 30. For now, just appreciate that starches, and fruits, fuel muscles involved in both cardio and weight-lifting activity.

Whether carbohydrates digest fast or slowly is an important concept in eating for health. Fast carbs generate more insulin response. Insulin is a «build fat» message in the body. Most people are trying to avoid that effect. Read more about this in the chapters on controling weight, triglycerides and diabetes.

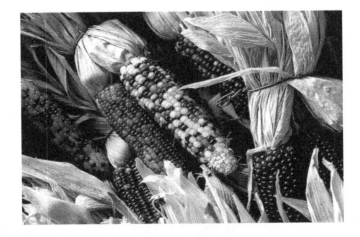

Fuel for your brain and muscles: carbohydrates

Here is a list of starches or carbohydrates. The foods at the top of the list are the best starches to be eating. They digest slowly. Eat less of the foods at the bottom.

Carbohydrates (starches) digest, and become blood sugar. Starches that digest slowly are the best ones for keeping a steady, supply of energy coming into your brain and muscles.

Legumes and (sweet) potatoes give you 3-4 times more of minerals like magnesium and potassium than do rice and pasta or even whole wheat bread.

Notice, beans are a starch! They have more protein compared to grains, but only 7 grams protein per 1/2 cup. They are the ideal starch. Try to eat 1/2 cup every day for the minerals.

"Eat more whole grains" says everyone. While these are better than white, processed grains, legumes and roots are much more nutritious.

Careful: more people get intestinal discomfort from white or whole wheat than anyone realizes. Try eating wheat-free for 10 days. See reflux remedies p. 95 too.

Black beans
Red kidney beans
White kidney beans
Pinto beans
Lentils
Chickpeas
Black-eyed peas
Navy beans
Lima beans
Humus

Sweet potatoes
Yams
Peas
Corn
Buckwheat
Plantain
White potatoes

Barley
Quinoa
Soba Noodles
Oatmeal
Cheerios
Buckwheat cereals
Corn tortillas
100% Rye bread
Brown rice

careful
Whole wheat bread
Spaghetti/noodles
White bread
Bagels
Rice
Saltines
Muffins
Waffles
Pancakes

Cookies
Cakes
Candy

Be careful in picking your starches

Sunlight beams down energy, linking carbon and water together, forming carbohydrates: hydrated carbon. We eat grains, roots, beans and fruits. After digestion, those hydrated bits of carbon travel to cells to be used for fuel. We extract the sunlight energy from the food, exhaling out carbon dioxide and water vapor. It is a very elegant process. Some bits of energy go astray, and this is one origin of «stray electrons» also known as «free radicals». Cleaning up stray electrons is an important activity in the body, otherwise the charged particles cause damage: think of it as mini-sunburns in cells.

A bit of advice. Don't get too swept away in the low carbohydrate diet trend. Being careful of starches and carbs for a few months, as part of a weight loss effort is fine. The emphasis on significantly limiting carbs applies mostly to sedentary people with extra upper-body area fat (apple-shaped people) who are trying to lose weight. People carrying their extra weight below the belt, pear-shaped, should continue to enjoy carbs, and just walk off their stored fat. Eating a diet too low in carbohydrates for too long can slow down metabolism, meaning the body adapts to living with lower fuel needs.

Carbs/starches are important for helping maintain a good metabolic rate. Starch calories are also important for people who have a good fitness routine. After exercise, muscles need to replenish their glycogen (stored starch) calories, otherwise they won't have fuel to perform tomorrow. Low fuel levels leave people with a feeling of fatigue.

Some people do need to still be careful of their carbohydrate servings at each meal or snack. For people who have a «thrift gene», ie they gain weight easily, and the weight is in the mid-abdomen area, yes, watching carbohydrate does matter. Half the black women in America have that "thrift" gene[71] which turns any extra carbohydrate calories to fat quickly. The same is true for many Hispanic people. Also, if you were once obese, and now trim, you have fat cells ready to ambush you and make fat quickly. You'll want to keep your carb/starch servings to a size that carefully matches your metabolic needs at the moment. See the diabetes and weight control sections for more help with this; this info is at page 108.

Remember, when you look at the science of how the body changes with age, we "caramelize": sugars stick to proteins. You see the effect in browned foods, like the end cuts of roast beef. I mentioned the fun acronym called A.G.E. – Advanced Glycation Endproducts. Eating heat-treated ie "browned foods" is one way to end up with more AGE in the body.[72] When people over-eat carbohydrates at any meal and the sugars hang around, the system does more caramelizing, i.e. makes glycated endproducts. These are irritating to the body, and have implications for the development of heart disease, Alzheimer's and kidney failure. Research is now looking in to what foods, like ginger, cumin, and cinnamon may inhibit the process.[73] This is especially important in diabetes care.

You need to know the fats of life!

You want to think about which fats are the natural ones that your body is most comfortable metabolizing. The fats found in fish are important to health; in turkey and chicken are ok. For thousands of years, the fats in nuts and seeds have been the oils your body expects to encounter every day.

Modern fats, like corn oil, vegetable oil, Crisco, beef fat and cheese fat, are harder for your body to deal with. The easy way to picture it: Crisco, meat and cheese fat are thick and make you dense too. The modern oils, like corn and vegetable, are too thin: too chemically unstable even. Stray electrons can turn them rancid easily. In essence, they can make your system over-react to irritations. An example, if you have arthritis, the modern oils can make you feel more –itis-. If you have hepatitis, your cells can be more irritated from eating too much modern fat. Basically, the wrong fat and oils enhance the inflammation process that you are trying to inhibit with fish oils, ibuprofen or aspirin.[74]

If you are a person who already turns starch to fat in a hurry, eating more beef and cheese fat can make you even more likely to store fat. The presence of these fats in your system triggers bigger amounts of insulin release.[75]

The oils in fish, like salmon, sardines and herring, tell your body to try to burn off fat. They also turn down the «make starch into fat» message. They are anti-inflammatory as well.[76] You probably know the term for these good fats: omega 3's. They have code letters to identify them: EPA and DHA.

Again, think back to the good old days, 38,000 years ago, nuts and berries were the routine afternoon snack. When eating nuts and seeds, a handful is 1 serving. Remember, you'd have to climb another tree to get a second handful. You'd usually go looking for easier-to-gather snacks, so diet was not overly fatty then.

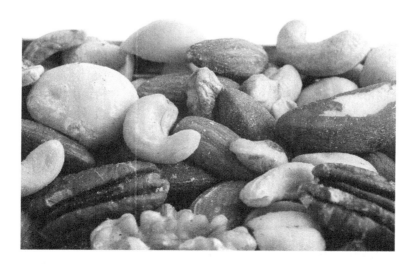

Caveperson fats: nuts & seeds

Fats that are still here from caveman times keep your body in good shape.

For a while, the nutrition message said all fat is bad. This was the wrong advice.

Nut oils and fish oils keep your body slick and flexible. This is good for keeping your blood flowing well and your brain thinking sharply.

Just imagine thick, stiff fat clogging the works. Air does not get into your lungs well. Blood doesn't get to your muscles as well. Brain cells are sluggish too.

Important: modern poly-unsaturated oils can cause excess inflammation. Avoid corn and vegetable oils.

Cooking idea: toss a tablespoon of nuts or seeds on your vegetables at supper, like walnuts on your spinach or pine nuts on cauliflower.

Fruit and nuts are a smart snack in the morning or afternoon.

Almonds
Walnuts
Pecans
Brazil nuts
Cashews
Pistachio nuts
Pine nuts
Macadamia nuts
Ground Flax Seeds

Sunflower seeds
Pumpkin seeds
Sesame seeds

Olives
Avocado

Peanuts
Soy nuts

Olive oil
Omega 3 butter

(*be modest*)
Smart Balance
  /tub margarine
Canola oil

 (*avoid*)
Cottonseed oil
Corn oil
Safflower oil
Fried fast foods
Lard
Stick margarine
Cream cheese

The good fats story continues ...

In nature, there are omega 3 fats in plants, like seaweed, purslane, and other leafy greens. There are omega 3 fats in pecans and walnuts and ground flax seeds. There are some in canola and soy oils too. All the plant forms of omega 3 fat are termed ALA, alpha linolenic acid. Only about one tenth of the ALA omega 3's that humans eat gets transformed to the longer molecules we commonly call omega 3 fish oils, labeled EPA and DHA, eicosapentaenoic acid and docosahexaenoic acid.[77]

I point out the difference, simply because all omega 3's don't act alike. They are all structurally useful, but it is the EPA and DHA forms that are much more potent when it comes to being anti-inflammation agents in the body. For instance, I don't want you thinking that the ground flax seeds dusted into your yogurt or salad will keep your lungs calm as a person with asthma, the way EPA/DHA in salmon, trout and fish oil pills will.[78] The ALA will not sooth arthritic joints either.

The fat that predominates in corn oil, vegetable oil, safflower oil, and even soybean oil and most seeds is the omega 6 fat linoleic acid, code letters LA. Like omega 3's these are processed to longer molecules in our bodies; most of them become something called AA, arachidonic acid. I only point this out because AA feeds the inflammation-generating agents called prostaglandins, like PGE_2 (pronounced prostaglandin E two).[79] People take aspirin and Motrin to stop PGE_2 – induced inflammation activity and pain.

A diet too high in omega 6 fats can result in excess PGE_2 inflammatory signal going through the body. Instead of risking side effects from non-steroidal agents like Motrin, ibuprofen and Celebrex which are all pills taken to reduce PGE_2 production, you can simply start to deprive the system of excess inflammatory oils.

Just a neat nutrition note, Andrew Stoll, MD, at Harvard University, is conducting studies where he is treating depression with 5 to 10 grams a day of supplemental EPA/DHA fish oil (in pill form),[80] and people's moods are lifting. (see www.omegabrite.com for info.)

Speaking of omega 3 fish oils, at the Framingham Heart Study, people eating fish three times a week, had higher DHA levels in their blood, and cut their risk of senile dementia in half, compared to people with lower DHA amounts. Fish plus other elements in the Mediterranean seem to reduce rates of dementia.[81] When I encounter people who are lacto-ovo vegetarian and simply don't eat any fish, I tell them I am worried about their aging brain and its structural need for EPA/DHA. I encourage them to either consume some fish oil pills, or look into the DHA supplements that are made from an algae source.[82] There are "gummy fish" style candy supplements that contain algae-derived DHA.[83] Taking 140 mg a day would be a wise idea. The risk of Alzheimer's disease goes up in people with lower levels of DHA in the brain,[84] as does the risk of decline in eyesight.[85]

A wonderful psychiatric researcher at NIH, Joseph Hibbeln MD, lectures on the topic of EPA/DHA deficiency and development of chronic disease. He has looked at fish consumption in various countries and the assortment of health problems that develop. He points out that in Japan, about the highest EPA/DHA consumption country, heart disease, stroke, and depression rates are radically lower than places like the USA or even Poland.[86] Dr. Hibbeln, in medical articles, also talks about the imbalance of Omega 6 and omega 3 levels in our American diet, and the resulting higher incidence of dyslexia, of hyperactivity disorders and even of tendency to violence. He also cited a 2002 study showing that adding vitamins, minerals and omega 3 fatty acids to young adult British prisoners' diets reduced antisocial behavioral offenses by 37 percent in nine months.[87]

The nutrition science and metabolic concept to carry with you is that all cells in the body have a fat component to the membrane wall. How the cell operates, then, is a function of cell wall fat composition. A better omega 3 fat component of the wall has a beneficial impact on so many conditions. The list includes hypertension, heart disease, diabetes, arthritis, anxiety and depression.[88]

At the time of this writing, there is a growing movement for the use of (food-grade) coconut oil to also help brain activity. The lauric acid, a 10-carbon fatty acid, found there, can be a fuel for brain cells, clogged with the plaques of Alzheimers. There are no science intervention studies that prove benefit, or possible risks. There is much wrong information that says the saturated fat of coconut oil is unhealthy. It is not. It leaves bad cholesterol alone, and raises good/ HDL cholesterol. Look for Mary Enig Ph.D. publications on the Internet. Two teaspoons a day could be useful.

Your body evolved expecting you to be eating the oils found in fish, sometimes from birds, and maybe a little fat from a swift, lean animal. Toss in some nuts and seeds, and you get the full picture of the fats your ancestors experienced. Your brain cells especially want you eating essential EPA/DHA omega 3 fats.

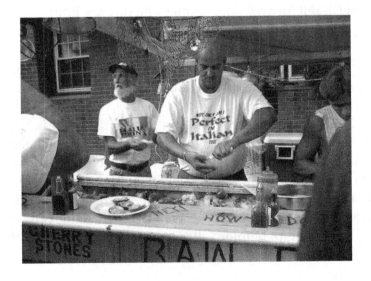

The Right Amount Of Food: understanding fuel needs

As you would imagine, genes, personality and lifestyle elements all contribute to your fuel needs. The response to stress is usually weight accumulation. The response to sleep deprivation is usually weight accumulation. Genes play a role in metabolism, but it's too late to pick new parents. You likely already have a sense of whether you have a slow or faster metabolism, as dictated by genetics. There is a section on weight control, starting at page 85, that may help people who struggle with weight management.

For now, think of fuel in two segments. There is energy you need to repair and restore your basic core self. This is the energy for your heart, your brain, your kidneys, your intestines, your liver and basic systems: your basal metabolism. Then you want to think about fuel for the physical activity aspect of life. Obviously, different people have differing activity levels. Ballroom dance and yoga classes don't require as much fuel as what you would need for your daily, hour-long, jogging, swimming and cycling sessions.

Various body parts have different fuel needs. The brain runs on sugar. The heart runs on fats. The diaphragm runs on a mixture: half fat and half sugar. Arm and leg muscles run on a mixture that is about 80% starch and 20% fat, in general. For active people, you may like to know that after about 25 minutes of continuous aerobic effort, the arm and leg fuel mix can change, burning more like 50% to 60% fat. Just so you know, the fuel mix change happens after 10 or 20 minutes in earlier years; this is part of what makes weight control harder as people age.

An average metabolism for a person over 50, can be about 13 to 15 calories per pound of ideal weight. We all know a few people that seem to eat tons of food, and stay amazingly thin. They are not the average person. The 13-15 calories number presumes that you are doing some modest physical movement each day, like housecleaning, walking 10 minutes to the bus stop and back each day, and maybe some occasional yard work. Add on the fuel needs of either coping with HIV infection, or of taking anti-HIV meds, and you figure another 1-2 calories per pound of what you weight. You could guesstimate that 14- 17 calories per pound of ideal weight is a good figure to start with.

At the age of 55 and older, your metabolic systems may be slowing down. If you have a thyroid problem, your metabolism may be slower. If you've had multiple injuries, and are slowed up, you have to eat a little less. Some medicines also make the body convert food to fat more readily. Some people think of type 2 diabetes as evidence of a thrift gene, sending fuel to storage more readliy. You may have to adjust the calorie level down one or two points because of these conditions.

More Physical Activity Raises Energy Needs

Keeping yourself in good physical health is one of the more pro-active things you could do as you age. Think about it: your heart pumps stronger, and the extra blood flow delivers more oxygen and nutrients to the nooks and crannies of your body. More antioxidants arrive with the flow as well. Doing 30 minutes of physical activity almost daily is a key component of mental and physical wellbeing. It is a good move to help feel more confident that you'll maintain good health in your later years.

If you are living an active lifestyle, give yourself some extra fuel when you do more workouts. On a Sunday, a two-hour bike ride might burn up 600 - 800 - 1000 calories, depending on your pace and intensity. So when you think of your total fuel needs, let's say you think of your core 160 lb. self, needing 2400 calories (160 x 15) and then you add on 600 calories for your 2 hour ride; you could eat up to 3000 calories, so that you'll feel restored the next day. This is not a "must eat" message, but I mention it for people who may be trying to do more exercise on a consistent basis, and I want them to repair and energize adequately each day. See the weight control section for how to cut back on calories when still doing a good amount of physical activity.

Also, understand what your body is using for fuel when you are exercising. When pedalling or brisk walking, you start out burning about 80% glycogen (starch) and 20% triglyceride (fat) in your muscles, but once warmed up, the mix is about 50-50. The fuel shift occurs about 25 minutes into the activity. If you want to eat some extra bread and pasta, exercise a bit longer before the meal, then there will be room, for the carbs in your muscles, otherwise the carbs get converted to fat. See the weight control section for more details about this.

Fuel Mix in Cardiovascular Athletic Activities

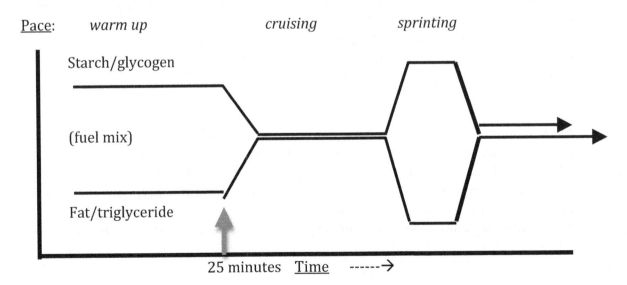

How Many Calories You Will Need Each Day ... (cont.)

When thinking about eating starches, a big focus is on how the hormone insulin responds. Insulin is a "move sugar" message in the body, telling cells to open up and let sugar, a product of digested starches, fruits and juices, into muscles where the carbs are needed for fuel. Insulin also has "build fat", "retain sodium", and "make hungry" messages. If you are working on weight loss, or managing blood fats / triglycerides, clearly you want to keep insulin messages lower. Warm muscles need less insulin to process sugars. If you worry about weight, and have the urge to eat some extra cereal, potatoes or pasta, eat these extra carbs after your brisk walk or bike ride. There is room in the muscles for the carb calories, plus there won't be as much "build fat" insulin message, sending the carbs to fat cells.

An important component of your daily fuel needs is dictated by your muscle mass. As people age, they may do less physical activity and their muscles shrink in volume, as well as strength. Doing some weight-lifting style activity is important to maintaining muscle volume. Bill Evans' book *Biomarkers*,[89] looks at how keeping in shape effects your «biological age». It is a great read on the topic of feeling and acting younger (physically) as our years advance.

Eating enough protien also matters to muscle integrity. Subtle deficiencies in protein over some years can lead a substantial loss in muscle cell volume: sarcopenia. The muscles may only appear to have shrunk a bit in size, but what has also taken place is that fats have replaced proteins inside muscle tissue, so there is much less strength. There will also be a change in fuel requirements. Fat is low maintenance stuff; proteinaceous muscle fibers need more fuel and nutrients to stay functional. Maintaining your body's muscle volume means you get to enjoy a few more calories still. Of course you still want to be smart about those calories. See protein requirements about how much to eat, in the next section. The book *Built To Survive*,[90] written by Michael Mooney and Nelson Vergel, is the comprehensive manual for maintaining muscles for people living with HIV. This book has helped thousands of people get their body back after AIDS-wasting.

good to know about aging + the body

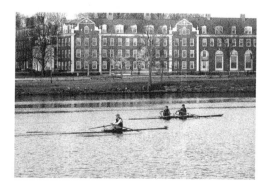

To decide your total fuel needs, think of your core body needs, then add on extra fuel for medical conditions, workouts or added recreational activities.

How much protein you will need each day

Recent research in people over sixty is showing that protein needs may be much higher than previously thought. The added protein is for maintaining muscle mass. You know about osteopenia, the thinning/shrinking of bones with age. Even more important, is "sarcopenia" the scientific word for loss of muscle mass. Less muscle means less strength, which can become a greater likelihood of falling, if a person gets to the point of frailty. Why and how muscle is lost with ageing is not clear. It may be the result of less capacity for taking dietary protein and turning it into muscle.[91] It may be that people are not using their muscles strenuously enough as they age, and therefore muscle mass dwindles.[92] By age 60, half the population is showing signs of significant muscle loss, and almost 10% have limited mobility as a result.[93] Also, the amino acids in muscles are the reserve fuel tank for the immune system. People can be visibly over-weight in appearance, when they have extra fat on them, but at the same time, the process of coping with fevers and infections can be eating away their muscle volume and putting their health in jeapordy. Jack Wang and Don Kotler in NYC were the first people to describe this situation in people with HIV, back in 1989.[94] They linked loss of body cell mass (muscle and organ tissue) with timing of death from AIDS.

People in caveperson times got about a third of their calories from protein.[95] Remember this was all the correct proteins; there were no other options. Even the flesh of grass-fed deer and antelope were nice lean protein, and rich in the omega three fats that we just think of as found in fish now.

After age 50 or 60, i.e., as the body ages, research suggests that people eat 1.6 grams protein per kilogram of ideal weight[96], which translates to about 3/4 gram of protein for each pound of ideal weight. The calculation: multiply ideal weight times ¾, to get grams of protein for daily needs. If eating higher amounts of protein feels difficult, then spreading out the protein intake to all 3 meals is useful. Remember, eating protein at breakfast is smart for your metabolism, and is a good way to be sure you'll squeeze in all that you need each day. It seems a minimum of 20 grams protein at any meal is what's needed to stimulate protein synthesis and prevent sarcopenia in older people.[97] Also, when working on the 3/4 gram per pound of ideal weight, having plant protein be a third or half of the allotment is also smart. This puts significant quantities of protein from black beans, humus and other legumes, plus from vegetables and from nuts, in the mix of daily food

A 160 lb. person certainly needs 80 grams of protein a day, and on up to 120 grams of protein is even better. Some people think, "Oh no, too much protein is not good for bones or kidneys or liver," but their thinking is out of date. Another idea to dispel is about eating too many eggs. In a group of exercising (weight-lifting) 61 year old people, raising dietary cholesterol intake from an average of 213 mg/day to 610 mg/day, by adding eggs, dairy foods and lean protein did not raise cholesterol numbers at all.[98]

Use this table to be get ideas on having 20-30 grams protein at each meal. Notice how nuts, seeds and beans can be helpful.

Protein Content of Common Foods

Amount	Food Item	Protein (grams)
8 oz.	Milk (whole, skim, 1%, 2%)	8
8 oz.	Soymilk	5+
1/2 cup	Low-fat Cottage cheese	14
1 oz.	Sliced Cheese	6+
2 Tblsp.	Parmesan Cheese, grated	4
4 oz.	Frozen Yogurt	2+
1 scoop	Designer Whey Protein Powder	~17
1	Egg, Whole	6
1	Egg, White Only	3.5
4 oz.	Salmon/tuna, canned	26
4 oz.	Fish, chicken, turkey, pork, beef	28
1/2 cup	Tofu	10
4 oz.	Tempeh (aged tofu)	17
1	Soyburger	10+
1/2 cup	Chick Peas, Lentils, Black or Kidney Beans	7
1/4 cup	Humus	6.5
2 Tblsp.	Peanut Butter	8
1/4 cup	Walnuts, almonds, cashews, sunflower seeds	7
1 cup	Broccoli or spinach, cooked	5
1/2 cup	Peas	4
1 cup	Pasta, cooked volume	7
1/2 cup	Quinoa, cooked volume	5
1	Baked Potato, Large	4
1 cup	Rice, cooked volume	4
1 cup	Ready-to-eat Cereal: Cheerios, Nutrigrain	4
1	English Muffin	4
2 slices	Bread, Whole grain	4
1	Sports Bar (Balance Bar, Power Bar)	10+

As you're thinking about protein foods, I want to emphasize how dynamic eating one serving of oily fish per week is. This could reduce risk of sudden cardiac death by 50%, and help people live longer in general. [99] Yes, a fish oil pill works too, if you simply don't eat fish.

Salmon salad instead of tuna salad sandwiches

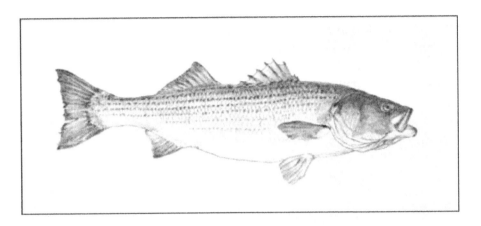

It is so important that people start to more consistently consume fish rich in omega-3 fats. Here is a simple recipe. Costco and Trader Joe's sell canned, wild Atlantic and wild Alaskan salmon. Skinless pink salmon, sprinkled with lemon juice, is as mild as tuna. When canned, it's lower cost, and no worries about mercury and PCP's in these relatively smaller, wild fish.

Instead of your usual tuna sandwich, make a mild salmon salad. Try this recipe to see if this is works for you.

Ingredients

1 6 oz. can wild Alaskan salmon
2-3 stalks finely chopped celery
1-2 Tblsp. Balsamic vinegar (Paul Newman's Balsamic vinaigrette salad dressing works well too.)

optional additions:
2-3 Tblsp. dill pickles, chopped
2-3 Tblsp. chopped mild onion
(optional) mix in ½ cup cannellini (white) beans and serve on salad greens.

Mix all ingredients and use instead of tuna on some rye bread or rye crackers.

These next few pages offer some sample daily menus to summarize what eating the right proteins, fruits, vegetables and legumes would look and feel like.

A food plan for someone who is 120 – 130 lbs.: ~1800 calories

Food		Calories
Breakfast		
protein:	2 oz. turkey, 3 Tblsp. protein powder or 1/2 C. cott. cheese	100
fruit:	a sm. banana, 3/4 cup fresh or canned fruit	80
nuts:	1 Tblsp. peanut butter or handful of nuts or seeds	100
dairy:	6 oz. no-fat yogurt or 8 oz. skim milk	80
beverage:	(optional) coffee, regular or green tea	
Snack		
starch:	1 granola bar, 1.5 C. Cheerios or 1 C. oatmeal	150
or fruit:	a small box of raisins or 10 dried apricot halves	
beverage.:	4 oz. glass of skim milk	40
Lunch		
protein:	3 oz. salmon, sardines, turkey, chicken or lite cheese	150
starch:	1/2 cup kidney beans or lentils or 1 cup peas or corn	150
veges:	2 lg. carrots, or a tomato and a green pepper	60
Snack		
Dairy:	8 oz. skim milk or 6 oz. low fat yogurt	80
Snack		
nuts:	1 handful (2 T.) walnuts, almonds, cashews, or sunflower seeds	100
fruit:	a lg. peach, 3/4 c. pineapple chunks, or 1 apple	75
Dinner		
protein:	4 oz. broiled fish, seafood, poultry, or lean meat	200
starch:	1 cup green peas, corn, limas, yam or baked potato	150
veges:	2 cups broccoli, cauliflower, spinach, carrots, etc.	80
oil:	1 Tblsp. nuts, 2 tsp. Smart Balance or 1 tsp. olive oil	45
Snack		
fruit:	a big orange or apple, 2 cups berries, or 2 plums or kiwis	100
dairy:	8 oz lite cocoa, 2 oz. lite cheese or 1 cup low-fat yogurt	100
	Total calories:	1840

(extra munch: 1 quart lite popcorn, 2 cookies or a scoop of lite ice cream   100)

Remember to be taking a better than average multivitamin along with this food.

Everyone has varying tastes, so these can be modified, and there is always a dessert cookie to add sometimes too. These are just the core plans.

A food plan for someone who is 150 – 165 lbs.: ~2300 calories

Food		Calories
Breakfast		
protein:	3oz. turkey, 1/3 c. whey protein or 3/4 c. cot. cheese	130
fruit:	a lg. banana, or one cup peaches, pineapple or pears	120
nuts:	3 Tblsp. walnuts, pecans, or sunflower seeds	135
dairy:	8 oz. no-fat yogurt or 8 oz. low fat milk	120
beverage:	(optional) coffee, regular or green tea	
Snack		
starch:	1 cup (ckd vol.) oatmeal, or 1.5 C. Cheerios or a granola bar	150
or fruit:	a small box of raisins or 10 dried apricot halves	
beverage:	(optional) green or regular tea or seltzer	
Lunch		
protein:	4 oz. salmon, sardines, turkey or lean ham	200
starch:	3/4 cup beans or lentils, 1.5 c. peas, or 2 sl. Rye bread	225
veges:	3 lg. carrots, or 2 tomatoes and a green pepper	75
beverage:	seltzer w/ lime or iced tea	
Snack		
nuts:	1 handful (3 T.) walnuts, almonds, cashews, peanuts	150
fruit:	a lg. peach, 1 c. pineapple chunks, or a sm. mango	100
Snack		
sweet:	2 fig newtons cookies, or 15 Teddy Grahams	100
Dinner		
protein:	6 oz. broiled fish, poultry, tofu or lean pork	300
starch:	1 c. peas, corn, limas, baked potato, or small yam	150
veges:	2 cups broccoli, cauliflower, spinach, etc.	80
oil/nuts:	12 cashews, or ~1 T. flax seeds , or 2 tsp. olive oil	90
	or 1 T. Smart Balance tub margarine	
Snack		
fruit:	a medium orange or apple, 1 c. berries, or 1 pear	75
dairy:	8 oz. skim milk or 6 oz. no-fat yogurt	100
	Total calories:	2300

Remember to be taking a better than average multivitamin along with this food.

Again, everyone has varying tastes, so these can be modified, and there is always a dessert cookie to add sometimes too. These are just the core plans.

A food plan for someone about 190 – 200 lbs.: 2800 calories.

Food		Calories
Breakfast		
protein:	3 oz. turkey, 4T. whey protein or 1 c. cottage cheese	150
fruit:	a lg. banana, a grapefruit, or 2 small oranges	120
nuts:	1/4 c. walnuts, pecans, Brazil nuts or sunflower seeds	175
dairy:	1 cup. no-fat yogurt or 8 oz. low fat milk	120
beverage:	black coffee, regular tea or green tea (optional)	
Snack		
starch:	1 c. oatmeal, 1.5 cups Cheerios, a granola bar	150
or fruit:	1 sm. box raisins, 10 dried apricots or 2 med. apples	
beverage:	green tea, regular tea or water (optional)	
Lunch		
protein:	4oz. salmon, turkey, chicken, or lean ham	200
starch:	3/4 cup kidney beans or lentils or 2 sl. Rye bread	200
veges:	3 carrots, or 2 tomatoes and a green pepper	75
dairy:	8 oz. low fat milk or fruit: 10 oz. juice	140
sweet:	2 fig Newton cookies or 2 small almond macaroons	100
beverage:	water or seltzer or iced tea	
Snack		
nuts:	1 handful (4 T.) walnuts, cashews or peanuts	150
fruit:	a lg. peach, 1 c. pineapple chunks, or a big apple	100
Dinner		
protein:	8 oz. broiled fish, poultry, or lean meat	400
starch:	1.5 cups green peas, corn, limas, baked potato	225
veges:	2 cups broccoli, cauliflower, spinach, carrots, etc.	80
oil/nuts:	1 Tblsp. olive oil, or 3 Tblsp. salad dressing or nuts	135
Snack:		
fruit:	a huge orange or apple, or 2 plums	100
dairy:	8 oz. skim milk or 6 oz no-fat yogurt	100
starch:	1.5 cups Cheerios; 1 cup oatmeal, or 5 cups lite popcorn	<u>150</u>
	Total calories:	2855

Remember to be taking a better than average multivitamin along with this food.

Designer Whey Protein Smoothies For Breakfast

Remember, the basic format for a smart breakfast is to eat protein, fruit and nuts/seeds. Since many people don't take the time to eat, I suggest they have a quick whey protein & fruit smoothie plus a handful of nuts, and let these be the meal. My Braun Multiquick handmixer is a great smoothie maker: $25. It's very durable.

The basic recipe:
Protein: 100 calories of Designer whey protein powder. (1 scoop)   (100 calories)
Fluid: use 4-oz/vol of yogurt or skim milk and/or 6-8 oz. of water to mix
       with protein powder.   (50 calories)
Fruit: have a nice large portion: a whole banana, a cup of berries, a pear,
       a slice of melon, a small mango, a cup pineapple or peaches   (100 calories)
Nuts: a handful, usually about 1/5 of a cup, of walnuts, pecans, almonds, cashews,
      sunflower seeds, or 2 Tablespoons of ground flax seeds.   (150 calories)
                                                          Total: approx. 400 calories

Examples:

3/4 cup applesauce	3/4 cup canned peaches
½ c. vanilla yogurt, & 6 oz. water	4 oz. milk & 6 oz water
apple pie spice seasoning	a dash of cinnamon
1/3 C. whey powder	1/3 C. whey powder
------------------------	------------------------
blend and drink	blend and drink

You can add 1-2 Tablespoons of ground flax seeds to any of the above drinks as a source of beneficial oils, or have a handful of nuts along with your drink. Raw nuts are best. Enjoy walnuts, pecans, Brazil nuts, sunflower seeds, cashews, almonds, and others.

Savory Vegetable Soup For Breakfast

A warm soup for breakfast is nice break from sweet foods. Some starchy fibrous vegetables can take the place of the fruit calories. Instead of whey protein, you can use a soy protein powder, or a non-soy vegetable protein powder. Peaceful Planet makes some decent protein powders. Their *Supreme Meal* is good for soups.

¾ cup Mixed Vegetables (carrots/corn/peas/green beans)
2 -3 Tablespoons Tomato/spaghetti sauce & 3/4 cup water
A dash of Basil, Oregano, Rosemary or other herb.
A scoop of soy or other plant protein powder (about 1/3 cup), dissolved in water.

Boil vegetables and tomato sauce with an herb for seasoning in 6 oz. of water for 5 minutes. Dissolve protein powder in water. Removed soup from heat, stir in dissolved protein powder. Eat as is, or puree with hand blender. This is nice for chilly winter mornings.

What About Vitamins And Other Nutrition Supplements?

There was once a popular saying, "If you eat a good diet, you don't need to take any vitamins." It is a nice thought, but no one ever really tested its validity. In other words, "show me the data". A number of studies now show significant depletion of nutrients from agricultural soils over the past 50 years, with a subsequent drop in nutrient content of fruits and vegetables, plus chicken and beef. Example, a 24% drop in magnesium content of a composite group of 27 vegetables in the period 1940 to 1991.[100] [101]

For the idea of taking added vitamins and other nutritional supplements, I use two perspectives. First, is there an element of the Paleolithic diet we are now missing, given how we eat these days? Then, is there a health consequence because of this? Vitamin E and heart disease prevention is a good example of both. We don't eat vit E as much as we did, and risk of developing heart disease is higher. Second, are elements of Paleo diet missing, and taking some supplements for a while could be therapeutic in helping repair? See the GERD discussion on pages 97 for an example.

In modern America, are we seeing examples of nutritional deficiency diseases? It is an interesting question. In general, we are not seeing much scurvy these days (a disease caused by lack of vitamin C). However what would more subtle, "sub-clinical" deficiencies look like? We think of heart disease as a cholesterol problem, or depression and violence as simple mental health issues. Some omega 3 fish oil researchers see them both as evidence of a deficiency in dietary EPA/DHA omega 3 fatty acid intakes, though.[102] In countries with much more omega 3's in their diet, there is not as much depression or heart disease.

Something about B-vitamins

A number of conditions do seem to have subtle nutritional deficits as a part of their development. Carotid artery stenosis, (the narrowing of the arteries in the neck that lead up to the brain), can result from modest B-vitamin deficiencies over time, according to research at the Framingham Heart Study.[103] In a survey watching 500,000 Europeans, better blood levels of B vitamins and folic acid seemed to reduce the risk of lung cancer by 50%, even showing benefits in smokers. [104] Just so you know, we eat less B vitamins than our ancestors did. Dr. Fawzi, at the Harvard School of Public Health won the Young Investigator of The Year award, from the International AIDS Society, for his work showing how beneficial a B-complex-25 supplement, that included vit C, was in raising both CD4 and CD8 cells counts, and improving pregnancy outcomes in women in Tanzania.[105] Mariana Baum in Miami has done some brilliant nutritional research in HIV+ people. Dr. Fawzi based his vitamin intervention dose on her work. In regard to B-vitamins, Dr. Baum pointed out that running low, or becoming deficient in vitamin B6 and B12 causes a drop in immune cell anti-microbial capacity, and immune cell count, and that it can take 6 months or more to re-establish the counts and germ-fighting competence after taking supplements to restore vitamin levels to normal range.[106]

The Case For Magnesium
National surveys detect that most Americans are eating only about 2/3 of the RDA for magnesium. This is 50% lower than the amount we ate in the early 1900's. [107] Might there be any consequence? Not many people are showing up with low blood levels of magnesium, but subtle deficiencies inside cells are associated with more cholesterol sticking to artery walls, i.e. more rapid progression of atherosclerosis, leading to heart disease. The "subclinical deficiency of magnesium leads to impaired bone calcification, speeding up development of osteoporosis. Low-level magnesium leads to more accumulation of fat in the stomach area.[108] I sometimes wonder how much of lipodystrophy effects could be attributed to lower magnesium levels in the body? There are only a few reports of magnesium status in people with HIV. In a heterosexual group in New Jersey, Joan Skurnick and her colleagues detected low blood levels of magnesium in 59% of the people examined.[109] In a German study, better magnesium levels were correlated with better CD4 T cell numbers too.[110]

Just an FYI note, drinking alcohol causes more loss of magnesium in urine. Hmmmm, beer gut ?[111] If you're not eating a half-cup of kidney or other beans, or 4 oz. of salmon today, or having 1/3 cup of seeds, you are likely to be not getting as much magnesium as is ideal. Seeds and legumes are not a routine component in many people's diet, so I like to see people take a multi-vitamin—multi-mineral pill that includes 100mg Magnesium.

Magnesium content of some common foods.   Milligrams

1/4 cup	Pumpkin seeds	185
1/4 cup	Sunflower seeds	127
1/4 cup	Almonds	98
1 oz.	Nuts: almonds	77
1 oz.	Nuts: cashews	78
2 Tblsp.	Seeds	70
1 cup, cooked	Soy beans	147
1 cup, cooked	Black beans	120
1 cup, cooked	Lima beans	81
1 cup, cooked	Lentils	71
1 cup, cooked	Green peas	62
1 cup, cooked vol.	Spinach, frzn, chopped	156
1 cup ckd. vol.	Swiss chard	151
1 cup, cooked	Brown rice	84
2 slices	Whole wheat bread	48
1 medium	Banana, 7"	32
1 medium	Orange	19

Magnesium RDA for people over age 50: females 320mg., males 420mg.

The More Vitamin D The Better
Another nutrient where diet provides variably sufficient amounts is vitamin D. Skin exposed to sunlight makes active vit D. Frequent levels in the blood have a range of about 20 – 56 ng/ml, or 50 – 140 nmol/L. However, deficiency symptoms show up at levels of 32 ng/ml or less, and <20ng/ml is very serious. Prominent researcher Michael Holick suggests "optimal vit D range" would be 50-70 ng/ml or 115-128 nmol/L.[112] People in the upper 25% of the usual normal range are maintaining strong bones; those in the lower 75% of the range are experiencing slow, subtle bone loss.[113] We most often think about vit D and bones, but it matters to muscle volume as well. The number associated with better muscles is 60 nmol/L.[114] The classical vitamin D deficiency disease is rickets, which is rare in the US. Meanwhile, other research data suggests that with lower vit D levels, the immune system is not working its best. Multiple sclerosis[115] and certain cancers occur more often in people with vit D in the lower parts of the "normal" range.[116] For many people, taking 1,000 units a day is the minimum suggested dose to reduce risk of deficiencies and disease.[117] "Osteomalacia is a softening of the bones due to low vit D intake. Let me also point out that the symptoms of osteomalacia are skeletal pain and muscle weakness. There are case reports where people complaining of painful bone ache went through the stress of cancer evaluation, because physicians don't think of vit D deficiency as capable of generating the pain.[118] Have your blood levels of Vit D checked as part of your routine health care. Again, >30 ng/mL is a nice, but >50ng/mL is likely better.

Vitamin D and The Flu
Vitamin D is emerging as a possibly strong agent for reducing risk of contracting the flu. First, notice that the flu seems to happen in the darker months of the year in the northern latitudes, and in the rainy season in tropical regions. [119] There is also data that shows people get more respiratory infections and the flu as their vitamin D levels go down in Fall and Winter. [120] Direct flu prevention trials using vitamin D have not yet happened. However, in several other studies where subjects were taking either 2000 iu of vit D per day or placebo, both anecdote[121] and data[122] show significant reductions in illness can occur.

Research on vitamin D for prevention of the flu is a big research topic over the past decade or so. First, let me point out that the true effectivemess of getting a flu shot is something of an unknown statistic. A quote from the journal, *Lancet Infectious Disease:*

Recent excess mortality studies were unable to confirm a decline in influenza-related mortality since 1980, even as vaccination coverage increased from 15% to 65%.[123]

... vaccine effectiveness, defined as the reduction in attack rates between vaccinated and unvaccinated population, expected to be between 70 and 90% in younger adults is considerably reduced to less than 40% over the age of 65 years....[124]

The vaccine seems do help small children and <u>frail</u> older people but only partially. Being older and frail is one of the reasons that the vaccine doesn't take hold, i.e. generate antibodies to the viruses it hopes to prevent. I mention higher vit D levels as a way to also reduce risk of flu incidence or complications.

Could better nutrition help a flu shot work better? That idea has only been slightly studied. A supplement drink with a basic multivitamin and some extra antioxidants plus selenium suggested there could be slight benefit.[125] Going as high as 200 iu vitamin E per day can improve the antibody response to diptheria, tetanus and hepatitis B vaccines.[126]

Fur, Feathers, Cysteine and Glutathione
One more example of diet being weak in a nutrient, with serious, but subtle consequences is the case of the amino acid cysteine. In the "olden days", we ate all sorts of critters, chewed 'em right up, fur, feathers and all. As a result, a caveman era diet naturally provided more of the sulfur-containing amino acid cysteine. Cysteine is the limiting amino acid in the production of glutathione (GSH); remember, GSH is the major antioxidant and detox enzyme in the body. GSH happens to support the repair of liver and lung cells. Glutathione also keeps eyes healthy, and prevents red blood cell damage from stray electrons, also called free radicals. Glutathione also helps insulin function at its best. Maybe most importantly, the glutathione enzyme has a lot to do with immune system regulation and function. When glutathione enzyme levels run low, the immune system struggles.[127] Many other repair systems also function less well too. Cysteine supplements used to be the remedy for bronchitis, in the era before antibiotics, but they still have a role to play in the modern era.[128] A large European clinical trial found that cysteine supplements, 600mg per day, was not of much benefit to people already taking steroids for their chronic obstructive lung disease. However, it was useful for people not medicated with steroids.[129] Well, people on continuous steroid therapy for lung issues should know that there is a significant increase in risk of cataracts as a side effect of that treatment.[130] Taking a cysteine supplement, like 500 mg a day, would be nice to try to avoid needing as much steroid treatment. The Droge group in Heidelberg has a number of papers discussing cysteine in HIV infection. They worry about low levels of cysteine causing faster decline in lung status for people with both asthma and HIV. They worry about cysteine deficiency in muscle loss as well.[131]

The reason I am mentioning cysteine now, is that better glutathione levels mean less health glitches in older people.[132] All the proteins we eat have a little bit of cysteine in them. It happens that whey protein is the best food source. Remember I suggested whey as the protein you have in the morning? Gut flora also produce key vitamins, and amino acids, particularly cysteine and L-glutamine.[133] So we're back to the importance of diet, and especially the fiber types, that will determine the resident array of beneficial microbes in the intestines (page 95).

This cysteine story illustrates an important point in this book. It also illuminates an aspect of modern medicine that warrants some precaution. Fast-acting prescription drug treatments for medical conditions may feel good in the short run, but may have consequences in the long run. Andrew Weil, MD points out in his book *Spontaneous Healing*, that people with arthritis who use non-steroidal anti-inflammatory agents for treatment, usually have a faster deterioration in joint health, than do people who make diet, exercise and lifestyle adjustments that nurture their joint surfaces.[134] We give antibiotics to treat an infection, so the drugs smack down the bug, but the body does the work of healing. How many subtle elements in the modern diet are missing and we therefore don't repair or heal as well, or our metabolism is not at peak function? Cave men didn't have fly ash and urban air pollution to contend with in their lungs, but if they did, they would have had plenty of cysteine to support the glutathione clean up system in their lungs. Today the situation is the opposite. More air pollution, but no one is consuming as much cysteine. Asthma rates are on the rise. So we know many people have lung cells that are struggling to repair, but they aren't eating the best repair nutrients.[135] There is a deficiency of antioxidants in asthma.[136] The number of Americans eating an adequate amount of fruits and vegetables per day to be nourished is 10% to 30%, depending on how the adequacy is measured. Actually, married seniors, men over 45 and women over 65 do better than most people, according to Neilson surveys.[137] Info on cysteine supplements to raise HDL cholesterol is on page 67, to help lower liver functions is on page 124.

Some Insight Into The Negative News About Vitamin E
One last example, of Paleo nutrition versus now, is about vitamin E. Cave people ate the equivalent of 5 or 6 bags of leaves every day, like spinach, chard, beet greens, purslane, arugula, etc. Between the greens and the couple of handfuls of nuts and seeds Paleolithic people ate each day, they got more vitamin E than we do now.[138] In modern diet, people consume only 8-10 units of vit E per day. Is anyone suffering from vit E deficiency disease? There is no evidence of deficiency diseases, but you might like to know that women with Paleolithic levels of vit E intake, about 100 units a day, in the Nurses Health Study conducted at Harvard University School of Public Health, reduce their risk of developing heart disease by one third.[139] A similar one-third reduction in risk of heart failure occurs in people with Paleolithic vitamin C intake, according to a very recent nutritional study.[140]

The point to appreciate is that super nourished people generally don't deteriorate at the same rate, as most people are currently experiencing. Medicines are frequently a balm on a wound that really would best benefit from healing support. Despite the rigors of living in the wild, ancient people had good health.[141] A web site with much, thought-provoking, information on this topic is The Weston Price Foundation.[142]

Anthropologists report that our caveman era, Paleolithic diet, was rich in vitamins C and E, and the minerals zinc, magnesium and calcium, plus omega 3 fats. They consumed these nutrients in amounts much higher than anyone ever eats now. Eating more of these key nutrients is associated with lack of diseases. [143]

The rest of the story on Vitamin E is in the subtle chemistry of its structure. Here is an analogy. You can have a left-handed potato peeler, a right-handed one, and one for ambidextrous people. Similarly, vitamin E exists as different shape molecules: alpha tocopherol, gamma tocopherol and delta tocopherol. The different forms have different purposes. Alpha is the form found in common supplements, and it has decent generalized antioxidant properties throughout the body[144]. Gamma is the "good stuff" for cardiovascular protection.[145] When taking high doses of an alpha supplement however, the gamma form gets crowded out, and the cardio protection action goes down. There can be detrimental effects of excess alpha and insufficient gamma on osteoporosis risk as well.[146] Consuming alcohol can lower good gamma levels too.[147] The bottom line is that when supplementing with more than 100 or 200 iu of vitamin E, be sure you are getting a "mixed tocopherols" supplement, so that you have the gamma tocopherol component covered.

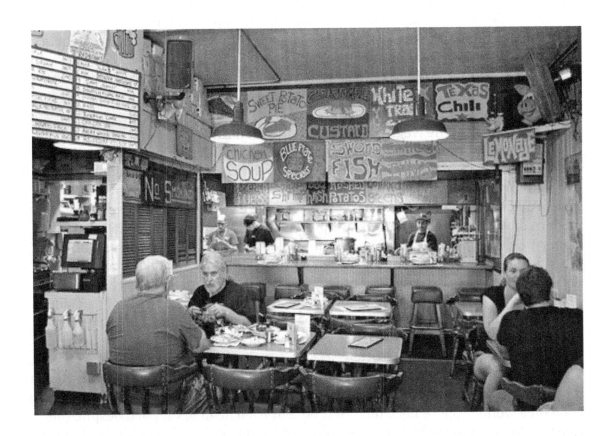

What would an incredibly nourishing diet look like?

The government puts out some recommendations for minimal quantities of fruits and vegetable to consume, to declare you nourished. These numbers don't reflect best caveman era intake, but they are a good start for supporting health. I list the number here so you can decide if you are doing pretty well, or need some improvement.

Dietary Guidelines for Americans, 2005
Fruit and Vegetable Recommendations

Population: Foods:

Women, Age 51+ years: Fruits: 1.5 cups per day

Women, Age 51+ years: Vegetables: 2 cups per day

Vegetable assortment to eat, cups per week:

Dark Green	Red & Orange	Beans & Peas	Starchy Veges	
1.5	4	1	4	cups

Men, Age 51+ years: Fruits: 2 cups per day

Men, Age 51+ years: Vegetables   2.5 cups per day

Vegetable assortment to eat, cups per week:

Dark Green	Red & Orange	Beans & Peas	Starchy Veges	
2	5.5	1.5	5	cups

Let me translate the numbers into simple behaviors you can focus on.

1) Eat a serving of fruit three times a day, meaning 21 servings a week.

2) Eat at least a whole box of vegetables daily, and then some ...
   One box of frozen vegetables is about 2 cups, or 11 oz. by weight.

So as you read this, what do you think? Are you eating the minimum amounts?

Your decision to take vitamins rests on several ideas.

Think about these concepts.

- Our metabolisms, operating on 100,000 year old genetic systems, are not experiencing all the nutrition that they are expecting, so our immune and repair systems may not be working at their best.

- Our systems may have some more modern metabolic needs than "usual diet" can meet.

- Your own taste preferences may mean that you are just missing some key nutrients in your daily intake, because you don't eat certain foods.

I would suggest that you ask yourself, whether your diet, as you eat now, is as nourishing as your body really needs it to be?

Vitamins are a great insurance policy for nutrient adequacy.

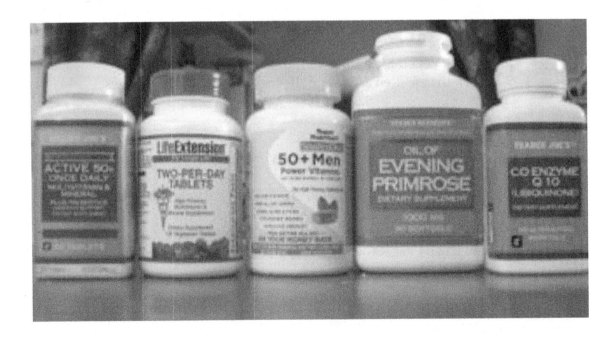

Should you take a multivitamin? I say, "Yes"

Think about taking a better than average vitamin each day, to cover some key nutrients. The term "multivitamin" has no special meaning; it just says a pill has several vitamins in it. When you are shopping for vitamins, CVS has a multivitamin, so does the drug company Glaxo, as Centrum, so does Bristol Myers Squib, as Theragran-M. They can have any amount of vitamin E, or vitamin C in the pill. They may include magnesium, but a totally useless amount.

There is a useful range of some key nutrients for HIV+ people to get when having a multivitamin-multi-mineral supplement. A vitamin should have 50% to 100% of the RDA for all possible nutrients, like copper, boron, manganese, but should have some Paleo-era level of added support in some key nutrients.

Here are safe and useful levels of nutritional support, lower and upper levels of helpful range are listed. In special cases, vit C or vit B6 or other agents may be useful in even higher amounts, for conditions like shingles or carpal tunnel syndrome, but those therapies are for a limited time and beyond the focus of this book.

<u>Vitamin C:</u>   250 mg on up to 1000 mg (milligrams).
<u>Vitamin E:</u>   100 iu (international units) up to 200 iu. if not mixed tocopherols;
       400 iu when natural or mixed tocopherols.
<u>B-complex</u> vitamins, which is B-1, B-2, B-6, B-12 all blended together, as
    B-complex 25, or B-complex 50, or B-complex 75. (The vit B6 amount determines how the pill is labeled. B-complex 25 has 25 mg of vit B6.)
<u>Magnesium:</u> 100 mg on up to 400 mg
<u>Selenium:</u> 100 mcg (micrograms) on to 200 mcg.

I like to keep it all uncomplicated and efficient. You don't need to be buying 7 bottles of vitamins. As of this 2014 printing, here are a few useful products that are available nationally. Check out www.NewYorkBuyersClub.org for good products like the Supernutrition items listed below.

1. **Enhanced Multivitamins**: 100% RDA for usual vitamins, 100 mg Magnesium, 100 mcg Selenium, plus ~10 X RDA B-complex, vit C & E.

Examples: Item	Available at	Cost/month
50+ Men by Supernutrition,	Whole Foods	$20/mo
50+ Women by Supernutrition	Whole Foods	$20/mo
Active Senior Multivitamins by Rainbow Light	Vitamin Shoppe	$9/mo
Two Per Day Tablets* by Life Extension	Vitamin Shoppe	$8.50/mo
Active 50+ Once Daily Multivitamin & Minerals	Trader Joe's	$6/mo

(Again: www.NewYorkBuyersClub.org)
(Find a local store or mail order: www.VitaminShoppe.com)

Nutrition Can Be Powerful!

I hope that some more science information will inspire you to make even better food and lifestyle choices. Smoking, poor diet, and physical inactivity were the main cause of death for 35% of Americans over age 65 in year 2000 statistics. Clearly these are 3 behaviors that people can change.[148] These health behaviors have consequences. People end up with conditions that require the use of prescription medicines. Use of prescription medicines is rising. This may be for prevention of future trouble, or for managing current illness.

Separate from their anti-HIV drugs, people in America are taking more prescription meds than a decade or two ago. As you age, you could end up in this drug rush too. You are already taking some pretty heavy duty anti-virals. Do all you can to not add more drugs with dubious benefit. I see people put on cholesterol-lowering drugs a lot, and now osteoporosis drugs. I want you to have a perspective on how much they may or may not help you. Nutrition and exercise offer you 3 to 5 times more disease prevention benefit than many common medicines do.

Table of Prescription Medication Use.[149]

% Americans taking 1 Prescription/day

Age group	Yrs. 1988-1994	2005 - 2008
45 – 64	54.8	64.8
65+	73.6	90.1

% Americans taking 3 or more prescriptions/day

Age group	Yrs. 1988-1994	2005 - 2008
45 – 64	20.0	34.1
65+	35.3	65.0

All kinds of reasons exist for the leap in drug-taking. A higher percentage of the population is getting health care, and treatment is more aggressive, for hypertension, high cholesterol and osteoporosis. Meanwhile, many people are taking drugs for conditons, but don't feel particulary better, and the Rx items may not be dynamically effective.

In looking at prescription drug effectiveness, there is a term, «number needed to treat» which means how many people are taking a drug, for there to be some usefulness for a single person. Example: in the «Statins to Lower Heart Attacks Trial in Air Force people in Texas, 375 people with high cholesterol would be on the drug Lovastatin for 3 years before 1 person is prevented from having a heart attack or stroke.[150] Would you take a medicine if you had those odds of it being useful? Would you look for a more effective intervention to reduce your heart attack risk? A recurring theme I will mention here is that medicines are not as helpful as people think, and that while lifestyle moves are not as easy as taking a pill, they do offer far more benefit. Let me just mention, that diet and exercise are 200% – 300% more effective than cholesterol-lowering drugs for protecting cardiac health.

Nutrition Can Impact Rate of Aging

There is a wide range of how «old» someone looks or feels at a particular age. There are a few research doctors who look at what might be the reason for variable rates of ageing. Dr. Stig Bengmark is a specialist in supporting the natural immune system and how that impacts aging. One of his particular interests is how to nourish the set of cells in the intestines that make antibodies to infections: GALT ... Gut-Associated Lymph Tissue. The friendly bacteria that live in our intestines, and the dietary fiber that support them, are the nourishment system for GALT. He looks at what might get in the way of having a healthy gut flora population. Prescription drugs, like Zantac and Nexium, disturb the gut flora, and of course antibiotics and antivirals change the ecology system there. Smoking cigarettes and drinking excessive amounts of alcohol damage the population of good gut bacteria too. Eating more food fibers, like the pectins in bananas, apples and pears, nurtures good gut flora.

Dr. Bengmark is also looking at what food is doing to immune function and ageing. He is pointing out how the processing of food is really disturbing key metabolism events in the body.[151] His particular concern is how excessive heating of foods causes inflammation in the body. He studies how A.G.E (Advanced Glycation Endproducts) contribute to chronic immune activation, which speeds up aging.[152] Remember, glycation is a fancy word for caramelizing.

People in their 60's and 70's very often have a feeling that their medical conditions are just a fact of aging. They wind up taking an increasing number of prescriptions to manage the conditions they associate with aging. Perhaps aging is not all that it appears. I want the info in this book to help you consider whether your conditons could be somewhat reversed with a smart blend of food, nutrition, fitness and energy healing modalities.

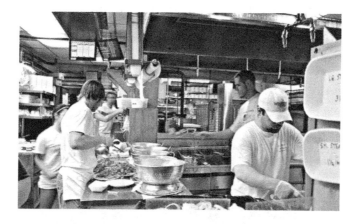

Holding Onto Your Body Parts

Medical Nutrition Therapy for Various Clinical Situations

The next sections of this book scan down the body, from head to toe, discussing aging, nutrition and repair. The medical situations and the nutritional perspective are detailed.

Once people are over age 50, many people are already taking prescription medicines they are not happy about being on. Others have some body parts that are not working as well as ideal. It may be higher blood pressure, or some finicky bowels, or acid indigestion. Cholesterol and or triglycerides can be too high. Crohn's disease, ulcerative colitis, and multiple sclerosis may start to feel worse too. A doctor may prescribe a number of medicines to manage these conditions, and very often people find the number of pills they take keeps rising, and so do the volume of side effects.

A smart program of diet plus some added vitamins, minerals or other nutritional items help cells function well, and the need for added medications can decrease. This generally means both better energy and fewer side effects.

The previous sections of this book have been about helping you eat the healthiest diet as we know it. It also outlines why you want to be taking a better than average multivitamin.

The next sections are to help you focus on areas of special interest to you or friends and family. The discussion is more technical. You may not follow it all, but you at least get the impression that diet and added nutrient supplements can improve your well-being. You have the sense that nutrition can help you function better and be less dependant on medicines that simply manage your symptoms. Now the solution is learning about what will repair the essential systems in you. You can take the book and visit a savvy nutrition professional to help you. As you have likely noticed, there are dozens of references in well-known scientific journals supporting the suggestions here. Show those references to the provider you are seeing, to add strength to your request for certain kinds of treatment.

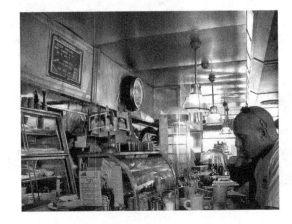

Feed Your Head: Brain Cell Support

Brain cell plasticity

Brain cell "plasticity" is a new idea getting a lot of attention. It is about preserving brain function through mind-body exercises. Learning a musical instrument is one of the best activities for this, as it involves conceptualizing thoughts, and muscle coordination activities. The brain has to open up new "passage ways" to make all this happen. It means growing cellular links. Up until recently, no one thought nerve cells could grow in adults.[153]

Dr. Herbert Benson, a champion of **mind-body medicine**, currently at Massachusetts General Hospital, in Boston, has stunning new data on using guided imagery and meditation to repair damaged nerve cells. A woman with a spinal chord injury, unable to walk after being thrown by her horse, uses guided imagery and meditation, to grow back her nerve cells, and walks again! [154]

It is slowing or reversing the general aging process in the brain that is on many people's minds. Here is a quick science lesson. The brain is composed of many nerve cells that must talk to each other. One cell communicates with another through a chemical messenger called a "neurotransmitter." The nutrition fundamentals are that a cell must make the neurotransmitters in adequate amounts for a good signal to happen. Also, the cell on the receiving end must be in nice shape in order to pick up the chemical message. So nutrients for production of neurotransmitters, and for cell membrane composition to collect the signal, are the focus.

Brain signal strength and adequacy matters to all body systems. Good flow of serotonin is an element of not being depressed and of sleeping well. Other signals help memory. Still others help blood sugar regulation, and digestion. The heart's response to stress, both the physical and mental kinds, again depends on brain signals. If brain is not at its best, the rest of you won't be either. You have perhaps encountered people who seem cranky and difficult in older age. It can be easy to judge them as difficult personalities, and lacking a loving perspective on people and events. There is a big biology to their behavior though. In Alzheimer's some people are experiencing less memory; other people have both low memory, are quite anxious, and sometimes physically combative. It is a change in cell architecture that is the cause. Remember, the cell building blocks are groceries.

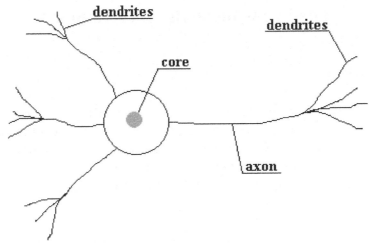

Diagram of a Nerve Cell

Too many free radicals seem to be one part of faster aging in the brain.

Fish Oils and Brain Cell Health

Many of the nutrients discussed as key components of the Paleolithic diet are key to brain cell health.[155] Again, the issue of taste preferences arises, and whether people are eating adequate amounts of key food items. You have heard that "fish is brain food". Cell membranes are made up of a blend of proteins, cholesterol and fats. Well when more of the fat in the brain cell walls is the omega 3 EPA/DHA type, brain cells work better. I have mentioned before, data from the Framingham Heart Study has shown that people consuming fish three times a week, and therefore having higher DHA levels in their blood and brain cells, cut their risk of senile dementia in half! [156]

How many people truly eat fish 3 times a week? Government research data says 50% of the population eats zero ounces of fish a week. A bit less than 10% of the people in this country eat 8 oz. fish a week. For reasons of cost, convenience or taste, many people are not consuming much fish, especially the kind that provides EPA/DHA fats. As mentioned before, researchers like Colonel Hibbeln, a brilliant physician in the U.S. Public Health Service, would declare poor brain function not a sign of disease, but a sign of malnutrition over time.[157]

Taking **Omega 3, EPA/DHA fish oil** supplement pills is an important consideration in the case of vegetarians and people who don't eat fish at all. Technically, eating 0.6 to 1.2% of total calories each day as omega 3 is the goal.[158]

Supplementation at 500 mg/day of total EPA/DHA is a smart minimum to supplement. This may be 1-2 "fish oil" pills a day.

See the nutrient label on the supplement pills to see how many pills it takes of a certain brand, to get enough EPA and DHA.

This is a sample label from a **Nordic Naturals Ultimate Omega 3 Fish Oils** product. Notice the data is for <u>2</u> pills, not one. You can see how much EPA and how much DHA the two pills have in total. The total Omega 3's part of the label can include some omega 3 that is not EPA/DHA and does not have the biological activity that you want. Pay attention to the EPA/DHA numbers.

Supplement Facts

Serving Size 2 SOFTGELS

Servings Per Container 30

Amount Per Serving	
CALORIES	18
CALORIES FROM FAT	18
TOTAL FAT	2 Gm
SATURATED FAT	0 Gm
TRANS FAT	0 Gm
TOTAL OMEGA-3'S	1280 Mg
EPA	650 Mg
DHA	450 Mg
OTHER OMEGA-3'S	180 Mg

For people who know they have heart disease, getting a total of 1,000 mg per day of EPA/DHA is a better idea.[159] People who are lacto-ovo vegetarians are consuming the plant form of omega 3 fat called ALA, which gives them some cardiac protection, but they are missing this vital brain support. The amount of ALA that the body converts to the brain-active forms EPA and DHA is a function of what types of, and what total volume of, fats are in their diet. I am worried that inadequate amounts of DHA will be available for best brain function for people not eating fish. Other research doctors share my concern.[160] While not making an official recommendation to take supplements, Drs. Johnson and Schaeffer, in mentioning their Framingham Heart Study research data, point out that an average fish oil pill will usually have the 140 mg of DHA, the amount to consume daily, to replicate the amount received in the 2.7 serving per week fish intake that lowered risk of senile dementia.[161] Taking just one of these Nordic fish oil pills would be enough to be good brain fuel.

In many aspects of life, there is a familiar phrase: "Size matters." This is especially true for brains. As people age, their brains shrink. Brain size matters to thinking capacity; a smaller brain is not as good at processing thoughts. The brain gets smaller from losing its battle with stray electrons.[162] Failure to neutralize free radicals is much of the reason for inflammation. Inflammation can come from chronic illness, too. Interestingly, carrying excess "visceral (abdominal area) fat turns out to even cause brain shrinking in middle age adults.[163] Given the number of overweight and obese people in America, the potential future quantity of people with dementia is staggering. Achieving and maintaining a trim, fit weight is not easy, but if you are worried about memory loss in older age, reducing belly-area fat is a one risk you can do something about.

Many events all have a role in the number and fate of free radicals in the brain. Foremost, the amount of antioxidant capacity in the diet affects how the brain copes with the stray electrons generated by everyday metabolism. In its extreme, brain senility is labeled Alzheimer's. In this case, brain neuron function is disrupted by the presence of a plaque called Amyloid-beta. How does the plaque land there? A simplified explanation is that a bit of magnesium is replaced with a bit of calcium in cell structure, and Amyloid toxicity happens.[164] [165] Much research is happening around how or why this occurs, and how other nutrients, like zinc and copper can disrupt the process.[166] A fundamental aspect of Alzheimer's is inflammation, modulated by the chemical substance (cytokine) called Tumor Necrosis Factor alpha (TNFa). Alzheimer's is a bigger risk for people with other inflammatory conditions. So not only does size matter, stray electrons matter too. An example: accelerated rates of brain shrinking are happening in "healthy middle-aged" people with metabolic syndrome (insulin resistance), even without actual diabetes.[167]

Nutrition advice for reducing your risk of senility and Alzheimer's starts with the caveperson-style food plan already outlined here. Omega 3 EPA/DHA oils are anti-inflammatory, and do lower TNFa levels in people directly. When obese people lose weight, their TNFa levels drop as well. The quote below is from the Journal of the American Medical Association:

The Mediterranean Diet, coupled with routine exercise, lowers risk of Alzheimer's more than either diet or exercise can individually accomplish alone. [168]

Here are a few food ideas to accent in your diet. Follow the advice of David Heber, MD PhD, in his book: *What Color Is Your Diet?* All the colors of the fruit and vegetables in the diet are various wavelengths of antioxidant action. Other substances, known as phytochemicals, in foods like dark chocolate, acai berries, red grape skins and red wine also have free radical squelching properties. The kinds of fats in the diet also seem to play a role in brain cell function. You know about fish oils. Olive oil is also anti-inflammatory. Replacing some grain calories with some olive oil calories seems to be one of the healthy elements of the Mediterranean diet.

Some new research results from USDA Aging Center in Boston and other groups are exciting. Supplementing laboratory animals, and then people over age 60, with blueberries, strawberries, almonds or Concord grapes,[169] improves memory function in as little as 12 weeks! [170] The idea that eating some specific anti-inflammatory foods helps memory in just three months time is amazing.

I already mentioned the magnificent properties of magnesium a few pages back. Here is yet another reason to pay attention to magnesium: its value in supporting brain cells. Magnesium as a food mineral plays a role in over 100 body chemistry reactions: brain cell construction and function included. Much of magnesium activity is helping squelch free radicals so there is less inflammation.[171] Remember magnesium is a nutrient at risk for adequacy already in the US population, especially older people. Similar at risk adequacy goes for zinc. Like magnesium, zinc matters to systems that repair proteins and squelch inflammation, especially in the nervous system. [172] This just comes back to being sure the multivitamin/mineral pill you take includes 100mg of magnesium and 15mg of zinc, as brain health insurance.

A vitamin supplement for brain cell support could be important for another reason. Homocysteine (HCYS) and methylmalonic acid (MMA) are substances that also irritate the brain and are part of the aging process. When blood levels of HCYS and MMA are higher than ideal, it is usually a sign that B-vitamins are running low in the body. A study of several hundred older people, who had normal B-complex vitamin levels in their blood, still saw elevated numbers for HCYS and MMA drop to normal in about ¾ of cases in 5 to 12 days, when given 1mg B12, 1 mg Folic Acid, and 5 mg vit B6. [173] These supplemented vitamin amounts are not much different than the common "Stress Tab" B-complex vitamin sold in pharmacies across the country. Part of the issue is, "normal" blood tests for vit B12 are a controversy.[174] Another aspect is whether the RDA for people over 50 needs some adjusting. While those debates lumber along, what you want to be looking at is the simple fact, outlined in the publically available article: *Homocysteine-lowering by B vitamins slows the rate of accelerated brain atrophy in mild cognitive impairment: a randomized controlled trial.* [175] Various studies place the number of people with low vit B 12 levels at a minimum of 15% of the population. Others suggest the number may be higher for people taking medicines that reduce stomach acid production. The drug Omeprazole can reduce B12 absorption by 66% or more, depending on dose. [176]

How are your B-12 numbers? In the Tufts Medical School *Nutrition For Healthy Living Study*, following 671 HIV+ people, vitamin B-12 levels were deficient or borderline-deficient in 22.5% of the people surveyed.[177] This number may be a bit high; that was the Viracept era, when diarrhea was common. However, something about protease inhibitor (PI) therapy causes just 10% of dietary vit B-12 to make it into the blood stream.[178] Dr. Margo Woods at Tufts urges everyone with HIV to monitor their B-12 levels, whether taking protease inhibitors or not.

This all comes down to the idea that taking a Stress Tab level of B-complex vitamins (3-5 times the RDA) is a good idea with no risk of adverse events. Some people monitor their Homocysteine for concerns about cardiac health. I suggest that watching it for brain wellness is a much more clinically useful reason.

One other aspect of brain chemistry and mood I want to point out. Depression is not just about serotonin, and taking Prozac or Seroquil, though. At best, about 10-20 % of people experience benefit from SSRI drugs. Actually, a recent paper reviewing all SSRI drug trials showed absolutely no benefit to the drugs, when compared to placebo![179] There are other chemical events at work in the brain of people with lower mood. It is a complex interplay of chemicals, inflammation, and blend of neurotransmitters that is operative. [180] [181] [182] James Gordon, MD wrote a wonderful book, called *Unstuck*, to help people with depression. This progressive psychiatrist is very clear and detailed about how little benefit depression drugs provide, and how they damage brain cells over time. He advocates using meds a bit to get a lift, but then details diet, vitamins, exercise and mental perspectives to really address the problem.[183]

I want to make one other point about mood. The Life Extension Foundation (lef.org) magazine featured an article several years ago, called *The Chemistry of Calm.* There is a book by the same name, by Henry Emmons, MD. The doctor points out that many people have a persistent anxiety that wears them out and they then get depressed. When I present this concept to many of my patients, it does resonate with them. What I also like about Dr. Emmons approach is that he advocates nutritional intervention ahead of drugs.[184] He often recommends the taking of EPA/DHA omega 3 fish oils, and B-complex vitamins. Among the additional supplements he mentions is the glutathione-supportive amino acid NAC/N-acetylcysteine, for its calming effect in the hypothalamus (forebrain). This nutrient has great utility in lungs, liver and kidneys of people with HIV, acting through its glutathione support. Again, excessive inflammation is not good in any body parts, including in the brain.

I hate to sound dark and dismal, but here goes. About 50% of America has swollen fat cells. These are a source of inflammatory cytokines and other rabble-rousing chemicals. As the population ages, and the percent of obese people rises, the horde of brain-challenged people will be staggering. How society and the medical system will cope with the amazing volume of senile people is unknown. The dollar cost alone will be staggering. Don't get caught up in the tidal wave. It won't be fun or pretty being in the flotilla. Look at food, fitness and supplements as your best hedge against a future with a dim brain. If you are reading this, chances are you take nutrition seriously. Talk to your friends. You may not have much influence on their weight, but antioxidant vitamins and fish oil pills make great birthday gifts, hostess presents and stocking stuffers. Show people you care; squelch their free radicals!

I also want to point out the value of cholesterol to brain health. I think there is a general idea that lower cholesterol numbers are always better, but there is a concept of too low. Total cholesterol at 175 mg/dl can start to be associated with depression.[185] Cholesterol in the 90 – 130 mg/dl is cause for alarm, says psychiatrist James Greenblatt, MD, of Walden Behavioral Care, Waltham MA, citing studies where anxiety and violence rise, besides incidence of depression.[186] Cholesterol is important brain cell cushioning material.

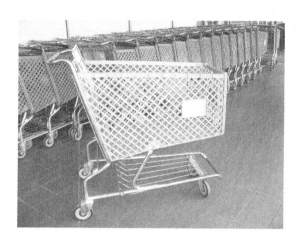

Cholesterol and Vascular Disease

The heart, arteries and veins form the cardiovascular system. In one sense, the system is simply a pump and the network of pipes that carries blood, oxygen, nutrients and debris to and from all the parts of the body. Arteries and veins are talented; they flex, expand and contract on demand, depending on the need for more circulation to some place in a hurry. If pipes corrode internally, flow is diminished. In aging, the system also loses its ability to be as flexible as needed. You likely know the term, "hardening of the arteries". As you can imagine, basic flow and flexibility properties are declining when hardening happens.

A plaque, generally containing calcium and cholesterol, constitutes the corrosive material in walls of the arteries. Simply, the interior diameter of the pipes becomes smaller: less flow capacity. With the plaque there, the endothelium (the cells lining the arteries) doesn't function correctly. For instance, the artery walls may not let cholesterol molecules pass through them, out of the blood and on into other tissues, so well. Arteries may accidently contract, when they were supposed to relax: something called endothelial dysfunction. When the very fine blood vessels of the heart become corroded, the cardiac cells are at risk for lack of oxygen. When a bit of plaque breaks off some artery wall and blocks a heart blood vessel, you get heart attack. Heart (muscle) cells deprived of oxygen hurt, and die rapidly. With age and other stresses, the cardiovascular plumbing system can become corroded.

The heart is a very sensitive muscle; its cells damage quickly and easily.

How arteries corrode, and the consequences.

In the diagram below you see an artery. Notice the artery has cells on the inner lining, and has a muscle layer. There are pores in the lining. When something, like "oxidized cholesterol" falls into the pore, it festers, and immune CD36 cells come to bat clean up. There is an inflammatory response for a while, and while things all settle down after cleaning up, there is a small scar left. The analogy is much like an acne pimple. Something gets in a skin pore, some inflammation happens, and a small scar remains. Accumulated scars form the plaque in arteries, technically the arterial walls. It is hardly ever mentioned, but the protease inhibitor Ritonavir (norvir), and perhaps other PI's, seems to activate CD36 foam cells, causing cholesterol plaque formation at a faster rate.[187] When I talk about supplements later on, I'll point out that vitamin E could reduce this problem. Interestingly, the old nucleoside drugs D4T and ddI did prevent atherosclerosis formation caused by Norvir in mouse model experiments.[188] It is not known about what benefit a nucleotide drug like tenofovir may provide.

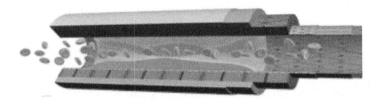

Actually, what gets into the cracks and causes the trouble are bits of "oxidized LDL cholesterol". Oxidized means this is cholesterol that itself has been somewhat nicked and scratched by stray electrons in the blood stream. Remember, stray electrons are the same agents that rust tin cans and car bumpers. They are electrons that fell out of their original orbit, likely at some chemical reaction elsewhere in the body. Antioxidants, like vitamin C and vitamin E and the color pigments in fruits and vegetables can tame stray electrons, which is why they are called antioxidants. You hear about the properties of red wine and dark chocolate doing the same free radical scavenging. In the past few years, there is a renewed emphasis on what is the real issue for heart disease prevention. There is the French paradox. People in that country (and Switzerland) have generally higher cholesterol numbers than Americans do, but they don't have as much heart disease. Many factors could account for their health, including a less stressful culture. One area of significant interest is the antioxidant value of their total diet, including the red grape/red wine antioxidant compound called Resveratrol.[189] In a sense, it is not the presence of cholesterol that matters, but how much "oxidized LDL cholesterol" is around. More antioxidants and anti-inflammatory compounds in the diet make a difference in the stickiness of cholesterol.

Avoiding heart disease may be less about having low cholesterol levels, and more about eating antioxidants. More experts feel that inadequate intake of fruits and of vegetables is a cause of heart disease.[190] Nearly 50% of people who get heart attacks have normal cholesterol numbers. There is much new controversy about how much cholesterol matters in general. It seems that high cholesterol numbers contribute to premature heart disease, but, in Framingham Heart Study data, elevated cholesterol is connected to all cause mortality mostly at age 40, and not at all at age 80. Cholesterol does connect to heart disease mortality at ages 40, 50 and 60. In an article in the Archives of Internal Medicine, however, the authors point out that *lower cholesterol is associated with higher non-heart mortality after age 50,* and that *physicians should be cautious about initiating cholesterol-lowering treatment in men and women above 65 to 70 years of age* until trials show efficacy or cost effectiveness.[191]

Some Cholesterol Controversy
The National Cholesterol Education Program (NCEP) guidelines say total cholesterol should be < 200 mg, Triglycerides be < 150, and HDL be > 40 for men and > 45 for women. LDL (sticky) cholesterol should be < 99, or < 130 or < 160, depending on age and other events in a person's health. There is much controversy over these guidelines, in part because people with significant ties to the pharmaceutical industry are the ones who set the standards.

A 2004 letter to the head of the NIH, the National Heart Lung Blood Institute and NCEP directors, signed by many prominent physicians, from Harvard, Michigan, Stanford, and Tufts Medical Schools, and endorsed by Senators Edward Kennedy, Judd Greg, Joseph Lieberman, Henry Waxman and others said:

> In petitioning for an independent review, we are not arguing that statins are not helpful for many people with elevated risk of heart disease. However, there is strong evidence to suggest that an objective, independent re-evaluation of the scientific evidence from the five new studies of statin therapy would lead to different conclusions than those presented by the current NCEP. ....

> While the latest NCEP report, like the 2001 guidelines before it, notes that lifestyle modification should be a first line of therapy to prevent heart disease, the sad fact is that these recommendations are being largely ignored, partly because the "experts," many of whom have conflicts of interest through their relationships with statin manufacturers, focus ever more attention on lowering cholesterol with expensive drugs. The vast majority of heart disease can be prevented by adopting healthy habits.

> The American people are poorly served when government-sanctioned clinical recommendations, uncritically amplified by the media, misdirect

attention and resources to expensive medical therapies that may not be scientifically justified.[192]

Lower cholesterol numbers are associated with higher mortality in other studies as well. A Honolulu group, based on data from 3527 Japanese American men, age 71 to 93, watched for 20 years, says:

These data cast doubt on the scientific justification for lowering cholesterol to very low concentrations (<4.65 mmol/L) in elderly people.[193]

Too low/unsafe Cholesterol?   < 4.65 mmol/L   =   < 181

Ideal Total Cholesterol	< 5.13 mmol/L of blood	=	< 200 mg/dl
Borderline high	5.13 - 6.13	=	200 to 220
High	>6.13 mmol/L	=	> 220

Again I will point out, if you have a heart disease diagnosis, you most likely need to be on a low dose of a statin drug. The effectiveness of this drug is less about its making your cholesterol count low, and more likely about reducing inflammation in your arteries.

If no heart disease diagnosis exists, a diet that gets your cholesterol numbers somewhat lower has many total health benefits. Medicines that get you to these numbers may not be of any benefit, and may actually have unwanted side effects.

As a nutritionist I sit with many people who are on high doses – 40mg – 80mg – of drugs like Simvastatin, Lipitor and Crestor. I cringe when people report these doses to me. They report a mental fogginess, and general tiredness, and wonder about their body sluggishness. When their LDL cholesterol is not at 70mg/dl, I can tell they are worried, like they are sitting in an unhealthy place. I show them an article from some University of Michigan MD's, a very expert critique of the LDL at 70 hypothesis. The title of the 3 October, 2006 article, from their Annals of Internal Medicine: *Narrative Review: Lack of Evidence for Recommended Low-Density Lipoprotein Treatment Targets: A Solvable Problem.* The authors are Rodney A. Hayward, MD; Timothy P. Hofer, MD, MSc; and Sandeep Vijan, MD, MSc. They simply point out that 40mg statin doses produced an effect of lowering rates of cardiac events. The low goal numbers were inappropriately extrapolated and the science of the studies does not back them up. It is a free article that you can download too.

Dr. Dariush Mozaffarian, a Brigham and Women's Hospital cardiologist, and Assistant Professor of Medicine at Harvard Medical School, is on an international committee that looks at Nutrition and Global Burden of Chronic Disease. Starting back in 2005, he was publishing information pointing out that **beef consumption** and **saturated fat** intake were less connected to heart disease than previously thought. [194] In recent years, he's even more specific that it is not about intake of saturated fat for heart health, it is much more about eating adequate fruits and vegetables as the way to heart health and prevention of cardiovascular disease. [195] If you have some time, watch his lecture on how it is actually the lack of fruits and vegetables that is a primary risk for development of heart disease.[196] A good study that proves this point comes out of Lyon France.

The Lyon Heart Study

Diet has a huge impact on blood supply to the heart. In Lyon France, researchers asked 600 people who were in the hospital after having had a heart attack to go on a diet, to see if it could prevent their returning to the hospital with another heart attack.[197] They placed 300 people on the NCEP1 diet (The National Cholesterol Education Program) asking them to eat a low fat, low cholesterol diet. They were to avoid eggs, and have just small servings of meat, chicken or fish. They were encouraged to eat more pasta, bagels and cereal: essentially the advice of the first Food Guide Pyramid. The other 300 people were asked to follow the diet eaten by the people on the island of Crete, near Greece. This island has a very low incidence of heart disease. People consumed more fish, seafood, legumes, salads, fruits, nuts and seeds. The Cretan diet has more carbohydrates from fruits and beans and less from grains than the NCEP diet. It allows more milligrams of cholesterol per day. It also has more fat grams per day than the NCEP plan, but the fats are from olive oil, a mono-unsaturated fat. The Crete diet also used a canola oil-based margarine spread, similar to Smart Balance®.

After 27 months, they checked to see how people were doing. Well, both groups had nice lower cholesterol and triglyceride numbers, and healthy HDL levels. However heart attack rates were radically different.

There were 33 heart attacks on the NCEP plan: 16 fatal, 17 non-fatal.
There were 8 heart attacks on the Crete plan: 3 fatal, 5 non fatal.

Let me say this again, so you really understand these results. Even in the setting of nice cholesterol numbers, there was a 76% drop in death rate by eating a more useful diet. Cholesterol numbers were fine in both groups, **food made the difference**. There is no prescription drug that is potent enough to achieve this powerful benefit.

At the 4-year point in the study, cardiac death rate is still 56% lower on the Crete food plan and there was a 61% drop in cancer death rates! [198]

The science concept here is that on a food plan with better fats and more antioxidant foods, your arteries stay less inflamed, and blood vessels stay more flexible. It seems that immune system cells work better too. Imagine: shrimp grilled in garlic and olive oil, tossed onto a mixed green salad, with some canellini beans in it for lunch, plus a snack of walnuts and grapes a little later, or almonds and apricots. Sounds like a tolerable lunch to me.

There is a shift in the old thinking. More studies are illuminating the point that the development of heart disease is not so much about avoiding dietary saturated fat and cholesterol. The real issue is that in people who do not have enough anti-inflammation compounds in their body, their plumbing corrodes with cholesterol plaque.[199]

Health status does still matter too, there are risk factors that raise the chance you get heart disease. These conditions all have an inflammation component:

Smoking   Obesity   Hypertension   Diabetes

Having high cholesterol or a high LDL matters for premature heart disease, but after age 60, it may not be so important. [200] For someone age 55 or 60 and older, it is time to be rethinking cholesterol numbers, and health status.

There is an incredibly informative book: *Overdosed America: The Broken Promise Of American Medicine*, written by John Abramson, MD.[201] He reveals the types of deception used in published clinical trials that get reported in medical journal articles. He explains the difference between changes in "relative risk" versus "absolute risk" in trial results. Here is an example. In the West Of Scotland Coronary Prevention Study (WOSCOPS), half of the 6000 men in the study were given the statin drug Pravachol, 40 mg a day. These men had average LDL of 192, and 44% of them smoked cigarettes. Of the guys on Pravachol, there was a 31% reduction in 'relative risk' of having a heart attack. This sounds great, but the 'actual risk' was much lower. As he says, "100 people would have to take Pravachol for 2 years to prevent a single heart attack." "In order to prevent a single death, 100 men in the WOSCOPS study would have to take Pravachol for 5½ years." OK, if you have a cholesterol level at 220, and your doctor suggests you take a pill to be healthier, would you take the drug, knowing that you have a one chance in 100 to benefit from it in the next 2 to 5 years?

I worked at the Harvard University Student-Faculty Health Service for many years. I attended many social receptions that featured fruit platters, along with cheese and cracker plates. One day, a doc and I are next to the cheese platter, and he said to me, "I suppose you don't eat this stuff," as he pops a few cubes of cheddar in his mouth. I replied that I do generally avoid cheeses since my cholesterol numbers shoot up quite quickly in response to just a few servings a month. He replies, "Oh, I am not worried, I am taking Lipitor," and then proceeds to munch some Brie cheese slices.

This is a well-trained, capable physician, whose thinking reflects the general medical perception of the dynamic utility of "statin" drugs in preventing heart disease. I want you to know better, though. My cheese-munching Harvard doc does not comprehend how little protection his statin drug is offering him.

The data for people who have already had a heart attack and are taking a statin drug to prevent another heart attack does show benefit. However, as you just saw from the results of the Lyon Heart Study, diet is still dynamically more useful, so don't neglect the food part.

Some people will do every possible nutrition step they can, and still have an elevated LDL. If they are reluctant to take a statin medicine, or cannot tolerate one, I don't want them feeling that they are in imminent danger with out the medicine. I want them to appreciate that diet is twice as preventative compared to the medication. I also want people to appreciate that exercise and fitness level are three times more potent than a medicine in preventing heart attacks. Also, see the vitamin E discussion later in this section and read about its help in preventing heart troubles. Also, there are some other nutrition tricks to do. A complete guide to lowering cholesterol comes in a few more pages.

The Details Of Heart Disease Risk in HIV Care

Understand Your Blood Lipid (Fat) Numbers.

Cholesterol is an important structural fat in the body. Think of it as the mortar between bricks. The blood delivers the mortar. There needs to be something cleaning up the stray mortar; that is the HDL molecule. Think of it as a dustpan. The other major fat in the blood is Triglyceride (TG). This is energy fat. A bottle of olive oil is actually a bottle of triglyceride. Fat and water (blood) don't mix, so Triglycerides travel with a cholesterol coating. The total cholesterol number you get at a doctor visit will include the amount of cholesterol that is wrapped around the TG's. The number that is 20% of the TG level is the approximate amount that the TG coating is contributing to total cholesterol. Subtract the HDL cholesterol too, now you can calculate the LDL cholesterol, the potentially sticky cholesterol. A doctor may decide to prescribe a cholesterol-lowering medicine like Simvastatin or Lovastatin based on the LDL number. Sometimes I see a higher cholesterol number alone being why people end up on a statin. Be careful, you want all the numbers.

Here's one other science fact to know. Low HDL, i.e. low cleanup activity, is seen as an independent risk factor for development of heart disease, especially in people over 70.[202] I see a lot of people with low HDL. This suggests that there may be an essential fat deficiency, or that there is not enough antioxidant action going on in the body. You can fix both of these conditions.

Normal Blood Lipid Ranges

Total Cholesterol	< 200 mg/dL ideal
	200-230 borderline high
HDL cholesterol	> 40 mg/dL males
	> 45 mg/dL females
Triglycerides	< 150 mg/dL
LDL-cholesterol	< 100 mg/dL optimal
	100 - 129 mg/dL above optimal
	130 – 159 mg/dL borderline high

Below are two examples of common blood fat numbers seen in HIV patients. Calculating LDL Cholesterol ...

	Case 1		Case 2	
Total Cholesterol		225 mg/dl		230
HDL cholesterol		42 (male)		40 (female)
Triglycerides	90 (**90** x 20%)	18mg/dl	300 (**300** x 20%)	60
LDL-cholesterol		165 mg/dl		130 mg/dl

Notice in Case #1, the total cholesterol and LDL cholesterol are high. I would always recommend a diet, exercise and supplement program to lower these first. If the numbers didn't improve, then the national medical guidelines say to treat with medicine.

Notice in case #2, cholesterol is even higher, but because HDL cholesterol is low and triglycerides are high, the LDL number is low. This does not warrant a statin prescription. You actually want to improve the HDL and TG numbers. In a simple way, the dustpan HDL is clogged with TG's, so stray cholesterol fragments are not being cleaned up. This high TG with low HDL pattern is a common marker for the Metabolic Syndrome. This means insulin is struggling a bit, and carb calories are not metabolizing correctly. Again, a low HDL means look for some issues with insulin resistance[203]. Earlier, common protease inhibitors, like Indinavir (Crixivan) and Lopinavir/Norvir (Kaletra) slow down insulin messaging, leaving sugars to turn to fats, raising TG's, invoking a diabetes-like condition.[204] This form of Dyslipidemia (a combination of abnormal fat levels) also suggests that sex hormone levels, like testosterone, may be abnormal.[205]

In HIV care, high Triglycerides and low HDL are often the more likely risk factors for heart disease risk; LDL-Cholesterol may or may not be high.

Appreciate some metabolism issues in the dyslipidemia (out of normal range blood fat numbers) of HIV disease, so that meds are not used inappropriately.

	More examples	**Calculating LDL Cholesterol**	
		Case 3	(on 10 mg Lipitor) Case 4
Total Cholesterol		225 mg/dl	278
HDL cholesterol		42 (female)	___? (male)
Triglycerides 350	(**350** x 20%)	70 mg/dl	1400 (**1400** x 20%) 280
LDL-cholesterol		113 mg/dl	incalculable mg/dl

You can interpret Case #3 now, okay LDL, but high Triglycerides (TG) and not quite ideal HDL. You can read in a few minutes about what nutrient deficiencies may be causing this. Case #4 is a guy I saw a long time ago. When TG's are above 700 you should really take action. The very high TG's can cause Pancreatitis, a serious condition. When TG's are this high, not only is the body producing a lot of fat, but also the liver and muscles are not burning up the fat/TG to make energy as they should. The mitochondria are the sugar and fat-burning units inside of cells. You may recall the term "mitochondrial toxicity of nucleoside analogues. This means drugs like AZT, D4T, ddI irritate mitochondria and impede the fat burning process. Too many free radicals, caused by immune activity also damage mitochondria. When TG's are very high like this, I caution people that stomachache and heartburn may be signs of Pancreatitis. If they feel those after eating, go to the emergency room and let them determine the cause of the gut discomfort.

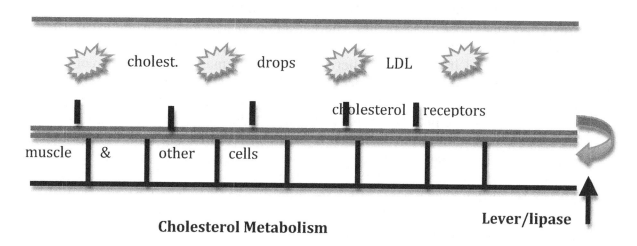

Cholesterol Metabolism

Cholesterol moves through the blood. The cholesterol droplets –LDL—hook onto cholesterol receptors, and a lever –a lipase—moves the LDL-cholesterol through artery walls on into cells where it will be used for things, like making vitamin D. LDL clearance from the blood depends on effective function of cholesterol receptors and peripheral cholesterol lipoprotein lipases (levers) ... the curved arrow in the above diagram.

There is no significant literature on the status of the receptors and lipase activity in HIV+ people. For any person, there can be some genetic reasons for who has higher cholesterol levels.[206] Separate from the actual cholesterol number, is the concern that immune activation, and the pro-inflammatory state, causes cholesterol to be deposited in arterial walls.[207] You can try lowering cholesterol with drugs, but I worry that while your numbers go down, your true risk will have hardly budged. This brings us back to a focus on antioxidants again.

More Attention To Vitamin E
There is a role for vitamin E here. It reverses the cholesterol deposition activity provoked by proteases like Norvir.[208] Before you get worried about taking vitamin E, let me review some science. In our primal forest diet we got about 100 international units a day.[209] Vit E supplementation seems controversial, thanks to some popular press coverage of some poorly designed review papers and lousy intervention studies. Women getting 100 iu a day through supplements, in the famous Nurses Health Study at Harvard University, reduced their risk of heart disease by one third.[210] Jumping to a higher dose, in the Women's Health Study (39,000 women over age 45) vitamin E therapy at 600 units every other day reduced the risk of sudden death heart attacks by 25%.[211] I will point out one more elegant vit E study from England. I don't suggest you try this alone at home, but I want people to know about a very successful vit E trial, that reversed heart disease plaque in people with existing heart disease. In the CHAOS study, there is radiographic data showing reversal of atherosclerotic lesions with 400 iu and 800 iu doses of vit E per day over the course of several years.[212]

So, why the vit E controversy? As I started to mention, back on page 43, the rest of the story about vitamin E is that it exists in several forms, somewhat like your vacuum cleaner hose attachments. There is a floor brush, and a carpet brush. The common form of vitamin E is alpha-tocopherol; it's a great general-purpose free radical squelcher: it does floors. There is also the gamma-tocopherol form of vitamin E. It has distinct and special properties, cleaning coronary arteries and squelching cancers in prostate, breast and elsewhere: so it's the vacuum attachment for the expensive import carpets. When studies give high dose Vit E as just the alpha-tocopherol form, the gamma form levels go down, and the body loses that special gamma activity.[213] Many vitamin E studies were poorly designed and gave negative results.[214] When it comes to taking vit E supplements, if you are taking more than 200 units per day, then get a blend of tocopherols. These will be labeled "natural tocopherols" or "mixed tocopherols". You don't want to crowd out the gamma and delta forms with too much alpha-tocopherol.

I emphasize the importance of still taking some antioxidants for the sake of arterial health. I have already mentioned the controversy over cholesterol numbers in general, and the issue of other places like France, with higher cholesterol numbers but less heart disease. I want you to not be treated for just a symptom, without dealing with the underlying processes: inflammation and oxidized LDL-cholesterol. Remember, 50% of people getting heart attacks have fine cholesterol numbers.

What was not fine was their inflammatory state. People without a chronic virus or two in their system may get away with the usual treatment, you are special, and deserve more complete and authentic care. An example, the meds of HAART irritate the endothelium, (cells lining arteries) and in the longer term, it seems this is a factor in the development of type II diabetes.[215] [216] We'll talk more about this later, but just one concept: addressing glutathione levels to limit the inflammation has been suggested.[217]

Low HDL is its own medical concern
The antioxidant story continues on to the predicament of low HDL. Medications to raise this are still in the experimental arena. Lifestyle factors, like low percent body fat and a healthy waist hip ratio and doing routine fitness activity all support a better HDL. Sometimes all these conditions are hard to meet when people are ill.

Niacin, used as high dose Nicotinic Acid to lower cholesterol, is the drug with the best efficacy for raising HDL.[218] People generally get 7 points rise in HDL with this therapy. Its effectiveness in reducing morbidity and mortality for heart disease stacks up well to statins. [219] One of the mechanisms of nicotinic acid is to improve the functional longevity of the HDL molecule. It also inhibits TG formation. It also has some antioxidant activity. [220] The European Consensus Panel on raising HDL-C is a good paper reviewing HDL raising strategies.[221] All the Niacin benefits it reviews serve the altered metabolism seen in people when taking antiviral medicines. The issue with Niacin therapy is that is causes a "flushing", hot skin feeling, for 15 or 20 minutes the first 4-5 days of starting it. Taking aspirin can reduce this, though.

In a subtle way, Cholesterol and HDL levels do reflect glutathione and antioxidant capacity[222], and healthiness of the liver. In the early days of HIV infection, the Droge group in Heidelberg was looking at the amino acid cysteine, and its support of the antioxidant enzyme Glutathione (GSH). They observed that GSH levels were low in untreated HIV+ people[223], and only somewhat recovered in people on ART, but still not up to HIV- people levels.[224] They point out that both CD4 cells and Natural Killer cell function improved when cysteine (NAC) supplementation restores GSH levels.[225] They also point out that **NAC supplementation, in the 1200mg to 3600mg range can raise HDL by 10 points!**[226] Just so you know, better HDL level is an important marker for reducing risk from cardiac events even into one's 80's.[227]

Remember this book is all about preserving body functions in the midst of aging and infection. The fact of aging is that restoration of glutathione levels goes on the decline at about age 45.[228] Now there is HIV infection and ART generating more free radicals, and a decline in antioxidant function. The good news is that the age-related decline in GSH levels can be modified by a simple amino acid supplement. Let me also point out that NAC supplementation seems to even help raise HDL levels and improve kidney function in people with kidney transplants.[229] People on treatment with tenofovir/Viread or its blend Atripla are concerned about renal function. No studies exist on what nutritional elements might reduce risk of trouble, but as GSH is the major antioxidant batting clean up in the kidneys, it's plausible to think this might be useful. Let me add one last comment to put NAC in perspective. In the pre-ART era, the Herzenbergs at Stanford University tried NAC supplements in people with HIV to discover possible benefit. The people taking NAC had improved glutathione levels, and lived 2-3 years longer than those not taking it.[230]

Here are two other fun facts about NAC supplementation. There is a long history of NAC trials in HIV care. Anthony Fauci, head of NIAID (National Institute of Allergy and Infectious Diseases), has authored papers on lower HIV replication with NAC supplementation.[231] There was a poster at the International AIDS Society meeting in Vancouver, 1996, from a Mexican group, which tried AZT-3TC versus AZT-3TC – NAC as antiviral therapy. People in the triple therapy (NAC) arm of the trial had a better T cell recovery. There is even more to the cystine / NAC story; I'll discuss it in both the gut and lung health sections. Meanwhile, let's get back to cholesterol management.

Therapy With Essential Fatty Acids

Let me tell you the fats of life. Dietary fats regulate many metabolic events in the body. Essential fat deficiencies can cause changes in bone strength, hormone production and even metabolic rate. In nutrition, we mostly think about omega 3 and omega 6, and a little bit about omega 9 fats as important. You see them listed in the chart on the next page. The omega 3 and omega 6 fats are termed "essential," that is, the body needs them for survival, and can't create them on its own. There are several omega 9 fats, the most common of which is the oleic acid in olive oil. It's a great, anti-inflammatory compound to eat, but not essential. No saturated fats are listed here. Those are not essential either; the body can produce them. Just so you know, when the body turns excess sugars and starches to fat, much of that fat will be saturated. Here is an interesting example. Cows eat grass and hay. When they turn any extra of those starch calories into fat, they produce the dense fat –suet-- you put in a bird feeder or the white fat you see on the edge of a steak. We're mammals, we make dense fat too. People that experienced "protease paunch" or "buffalo hump" -- the fat deposits from protease inhibitor therapy -- sensed how dense that fat is.

For a very long time, dietary saturated fat has seemed evil, but more researchers are taking a closer look at this idea. Replacing sat fat in the diet with carbohydrates, does not seem to generate cardiac benefit. Replacing it with polyunsaturated fats has maybe a 10% benefit. Interestingly, replacing the one saturated fat *C14:0* Myristic Acid found in beef, with the *C:12* sat fat called Lauric acid, found in coconut oil, has a healthy effect: raising HDL cholesterol a bit, thereby improving the cholesterol:HDL ratio![232] (The backbone of fat structures is a string of carbon atoms 8, 10, 12, up to 22 units long; hence the C:12 type labeling.)

Speaking of coconut oil, it has nice antimicrobial properties.[233] [234] Remember the days of Viracept-provoked diarrhea. Something about eating coconut macaroons was useful in reducing the diarrhea. I will speculate that it may have been reducing the volume of pesky bacteria in the gut. There is mounting evidence that coconut oil is good brain cell fuel for people with Alzheimer's.[235][236]

The Fats of Life

LA 18:2 *n*-6   **ALA** 18:3 *n*-3   **OA** 18-1 *n*-9
(corn/vege. oil)   (flax seed/walnuts)   (olive oil)

Delta-6 desaturase

GLA 18:3 *n*-6   18:4 *n*-3
(primrose/sunflowers)

Delta-5 desaturase

DGLA 20:3 *n*-6   **EPA** 20:5 *n*-3

Delta-4 desaturase

AA 20:4 *n*-6   **DHA** 20:6 *n*-3
                        (salmon sardines)
(PGE1, PGE2)   (PGE3)

LA is linolenic acid
GLA is gamma linolenic acid
DGLA is dihomo gamma linolenic acid
AA is arachidonic acid

ALA is alpha linolenic acid
OA is oleic acid
EPA is eicosapentaenoic acid
DHA is docosahexaenoic acid

Here is some detailed science on the structure and function of fat molecules in the body. I include it because I think it is interesting, and because very few medical people, including dietitians and nutritionists, understand the major degree to which fats regulate many metabolic processes in the body.

If you want to skip the science, then here's the take home message. You need two essential fat compounds in the body. Depending on amounts of fish and seeds you eat every week, you may want to take these supplements:

1. Take 1 - 2 grams per day EPA/DHA omega 3 fat as fish oils.
2. Take 1 - 2 grams per day GLA omega 6 fat per day as Evening Primrose Oil.

OK, for the science behind the recommendations, read on ...

Delta 6, Delta 5 and Delta 4 are the desaturase/elongase enzymes that change the structure of the essential fats **LA** and **ALA**, into other shape fats, with various functions in the body.

I describe the steps of fat alteration here, because they have many consequences for health. **GLA** is a potent anti-inflammatory compound.[237] Aging, eating trans fats, eating saturated fats, drinking alcohol and having diabetes all reduce Delta-6 activity[238]. Low **GLA** levels seem to be a risk factor for development of type2 diabetes.[239] Other chronic inflammatory conditions like eczema lower Delta-6 action too.[240] Leafy greens and seeds, plus some nuts are the sources of **GLA** in the diet, as is cold-pressed sunflower seed oil. I say eating ¼ cup raw seeds every day is a smart food idea, for getting some **GLA**.

A few important details about all this: if there is a lot of **LA** in your diet, there might not be enough Delta 6 left to convert some of the omega 3 **ALA** into the more beneficial **EPA/DHA** compounds. The Paleolithic diet used to have 1, 2 or 3 parts **LA** to 1 part **ALA**. Now, the ratio is more like 12-18 parts **LA** to 1 part **ALA**. The means food sources of **EPA & DHA** – oily fish -- matter even more.

There is no research data yet that describes **what the GLA levels are in people with HIV**, either on or off ART treatment. Here is an important story, though. Back in the days when indinavir/Crixivan was a common part of anti-HIV therapy, people taking it were complaining of amazingly dry skin, plus dry cracked lips, and ingrown toenails. Joan Connors D.DIV, RD, a very smart dietitian at the *Nutrition For Healthy Living"* study at Tufts Medical School in Boston, recognized the dry skin as a symptom of GLA, essential fat deficiency. GLA is the fat that is the moisture barrier in the skin. She suggested that people take 2 grams per day of Evening Primrose Oil, a handy source of GLA. Sure enough, in about 10 days, the dry skin was resolving. When people stopped the Primrose Oil, the dry skin came back. This was good proof of concept. Any of you who get cracked skin on your fingertips in winter, from living in a cold weather ZIP code, the two grams per day Evening Primrose is good to know about. The dry cracked skin on fingertips totally heals with GLA – Primrose oil supplements. This Crixivan experience has me forever looking out for signs of GLA deficiency in people.

Benefits Of Omega 3 EPA/DHA You Want To Be Aware Of

The omega 3 fatty acids EPA/DHA are known to be useful in promoting heart health.

> Simply consuming fish once a week can provide dramatic benefit. In the Physicians Health Study, heart attack and stroke events dropped 40% for people consuming fish as little as once a week. [241]

> In the 5000 person GISSI Prevenzione study in Italy, therapeutic fish oil supplementation at the level of 780 mg (combined EPA/DHA) reduced the incidence of sudden cardiac death 45% in people with existing heart disease.[242]

> Dr. Sherwood Gorbach's *Nutrition For Healthy Living Study* at Tufts Medical in Boston reported results of a 6 grams per day fish oil intervention in HIV+ people

with elevated TG's, showing nearly 40% drop in TG's.[243] How do the fish oils work? The EPA/DHA tell the liver to both make less and burn more fat.

Many people just don't know when they have "sub-clinical heart disease". Appreciate that diabetes risk, and a history of smoking, are significant issues in the HIV+ population. These, plus being HIV+ all raise the risk of heart disease.

My advice is to take advantage of the anti- arterial corrosion, anti- blood clot, anti- arrhythmia, and anti-inflammatory properties of EPA/DHA.[244] The brain support, anti depression and anti- Alzheimer's effects of omega 3 EPA/DHA are spelled out back on page 27.

Eat fish that is rich in omega 3 fats a few times a week. If you're just not into the taste, give serious thought to taking 1 to 2 EPA/DHA fish oil pills per day.

People with Hepatitis C benefit from Omega 3 fish oils too. See the liver section on page 124. Omega 3's help clear fat from the liver, reducing scarring activity.

Omega 6 – GLA fat benefits do not get enough medical attention

The omega 6 fatty acid "gamma linolenic acid" (GLA) receives less attention than the omega 3's EPA/DHA do. GLA supplements generate benefits in managing cholesterol, blood pressure, plus eczema,[245] rheumatoid arthritis and depression.[246] GLA is crucial to nerve cell growth and repair, and recently its value in treating diabetic neuropathy has been getting more attention.[247]

People with a GLA deficiency gain fat in the abdomen, and see cholesterol and TG counts rise, and HDL levels drop.[248] Sound familiar, as the common body shape and blood lipid changes seen in lipodystrophy?

The terms *Syndrome X* and *Metabolic Syndrome* both refer to condition where people are showing this lipid pattern, and a tendancy to higher blood presure. There is insulin resistance and higher possibility of diabetes happening. Read more about insulin resistance and inflammation in the diabetes section, starting on page 106. Meanwhile I want to emphasize, that higher TG's can be about essential fat –GLA deficiency – and that supplementation can improve insulin function, and blood lipid numbers.[249] The doses are simply two grams of fish oils, and 2 grams of primrose oil per day. There is no danger of toxicity with these, and many cardiac benefits.

So you may sit there saying to yourself, "I can take a few fibrate and statin pills from my doctor to treat the cholesterol and TG's, but you want me to take supplements. What's the difference?" At the risk of sounding like a broken record, I want to emphasize that nutritional deficiencies play out in many systems. Seeing high blood lipid (fat) numbers is just one symptom of the deficiency. Yes, you can take a fibrate pill to lower the TG's. Your next blood test will look good, but the fibrate won't alter the essential fat deficiency that your pancreas is experiencing, and will play out a few months later as a diabetes diagnosis. The fibrate won't fix the fat deficiency in your brain cells, which will play out as poorer ability to concentrate and eventual brain shrinkage. Fixing the nutrient deficiency that is behind the high TG number, will keep the liver, pancreas and the brain healthy.

The dylipidemia picture in HIV care is complex. Chronic inflammation, from the irritation of medicines, or simply from lack of adequate antioxidant activity leads to higher TG numbers. One other reason for high TG's is higher amounts of immune activation. The cytokines that direct immune activity, in a simple way, tell the body to keep more sugar and fat circulating in the blood, to be a handy fuel supply for circulating immune cells. This activation is behind the process of **lipoatrophy**, which is the loss of the fat stored in arms and legs, just under the skin. Again, a fat-lowering medicine will make the blood look better,[250] but you want the process of getting skinny arms and legs to stop as well. Too many stray fats in the blood, coupled with protease therapy, like ritonavir/Norvir, raise risk of cholesterol clogging arteries.[251] The bottom line is still to treat the problem at its source: in the absence of an infection, or a hormone (testosterone) deficiency, the inflammation is likely from inadequate antioxidant action, or from essential fat deficiency. Eat and supplement accordingly.

All The Nutrition Steps To Manage Cholesterol Without Drugs

First, the Mediterranean / Crete diet is what I detailed in the original food plan, back on pages 8 to 20, when I was describing the caveman time food plan. Eat that way.

Let me accent the important elements in the Mediterranean diet.

Key Concepts For Reducing Heart Disease Risk, And Cholesterol.

1. Eat A Lot Of Fiber: People eating high fiber (roughage) diets have lower cholesterol numbers and less heart disease and diabetes. You may have read figures. For women, try to eat 25 grams of fiber per day, and men 35 grams per day. Behaviorally, 3 servings of fruit per day, and 3 cups (cooked volume) of vegetables per day, (1 cup at lunch and 2 cups at supper) is the foundation of what you need. Then you need one other serious fiber dose per day, consumed as either ½ cup of a bean/legume food, or as a serious high fiber cereal: 7 grams of fiber per serving.

In the Crete diet, fruits have replaced some of the grain calories in the daily diet. This has a tremendous impact on some important metabolic events in the body.

Fruits are great fiber. Many people think they have a lot of sugar, and avoid them, and have a grain item instead. This is a mistake. Just keep the fruit portion to 100 calories and you'll be fine. Fruits contain a blend of fructose and glucose, and this mixture does not require as much insulin to process as would 100 calories of a grain. Fruits eaten with some protein, seeds or nuts will digest more slowly, keeping the blood sugar response lower. This is what people mean when they talk about "low glycemic load" eating. The rate that sugar enters into the blood, and the total volume of sugar calories, are both kept to a modest level.

Fruit fibers are probably the most important roughage in heart health.

FRUITS: Eat 3, 4 or even 5 servings of fruit a day. Eating an apple, a banana, or a pear each day is a good start, for a dose of the cholesterol-lowering fiber called pectin. Peaches, nectarines, berries and melons are good too. Dried fruits have fiber, as do frozen and canned fruits. One-half cup of peaches, pears or applesauce from a can constitutes a serving as well. Look at it this way, nuts and berries as snacks worked well for cave people, and will help you too.

Here is an important concept. Fruit pulp contains a lot of the water-soluble fiber, called pectin. This kind of fiber supports the growth of healthy bacteria in the intestines. These beneficial bacteria produce some small fat molecules called short-chain fatty acids. They have names like acetate, propionate and butyrate. These small fats are fuels for keeping cells lining the large intestine in good repair. The acetate and butyrate also go off to the liver and tell it to produce less cholesterol!

Acetate, Propionate and Butyrate, small fat particles, made by friendly microbes in the gut, travel to the liver and signal it to reduce cholesterol production.

Let me say that again, many people are eating a low fat and low cholesterol diet, yet their lipid numbers remain elevated. One issue may be that the liver is making too much cholesterol. How do you get the liver to produce less? Eat fruit, and have the beneficial bacteria in the gut make mini-fat particles named: acetate, propionate and butyrate. [252] These fatty substances travel from gut to the liver and "down regulate" cholesterol production.

Here is a fun fact. When you have stools that look like spongy logs that float in the toilet bowl, you know you have a good gut flora repertoire in your intestinal ecosystem. I tell people remember: "fruit, fiber, floaters". Asking people if they have floaters makes for great cocktail party chatter. Try it, you'll see.

Most people find that their stools float about 3 to 4 weeks into eating fruit more routinely. If this is not occurring, then take a "probiotic" (opposite of antibiotic") supplement.

A probiotic (supplement) will be a blend of organisms with names like "Lactobacillus acidophilus, Lactobacillus plantarum, Lactobacillus rhamnosus, Bifidobacter longum, and Bifidobacter breve.

When you look at the label on the probiotics bottle, the amount of ready to grow organisms is listed as **"colony forming units"** and a good threshold about is **3 to 5 billion per dose.**

I have good results from the product **JarroDophilus EPS, 1 to 2 pills per day.** Take the probiotic until stools float. Keep the leftover supplement in the refrigerator. If you see sinkers happening a few months later, just restart the probiotic pills for a few days.

Smoking cigarettes, drinking a lot of alcohol, taking anti-acid reflux pills, and experiencing a high amount of mental stress all seem to lower the friendly bacteria population in the gut. This may mean you need to take probiotic supplements a few times a week, to maintain stools that float.

Every once in a while, I will have a patient who is on an exemplary diet, and has taken probiotic supplements for a few months, and yet, poop never does float. I have no idea why, so I just ask these people to take 2-3 probiotic pills a week as a maintenance regimen until I see where their cholesterol numbers get to, on blood tests. Then we may try stopping for a while to see the results off therapy.

Many people with HIV infection, on treatment, end up having elevated cholesterol numbers. You have likely heard the old adage, that taking antibiotics kills off the friendly flora and people should eat yogurt to replace the good bacteria. The full effect of anti-HIV meds on good gut flora has not yet been well studied. The few research papers that have been published do describe an alteration in usual pattern. For people on a once-a-day ART regiment, like the Quad pill, Stribild, or Atripla in the evening, I suggest they take the probiotic supplement in the morning, so the good bugs have plenty of time to multiply. For a full picture of what is going on with the gut flora in people with HIV, see intestine section, on page 91.

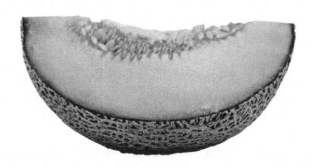

Vegetables are another important source of beneficial fibers.

VEGETABLES: Eating at least 2-3 cups per day of vegetables like the ones listed here is important to getting enough plant fibers.

Asparagus	Cabbage	Mesculin greens	Red peppers
Beets	Carrots	Mushrooms	Romaine lettuce
Broccoli	Cauliflower	Mustard greens	Tomatoes
Brussel sprouts	Collard greens	Pea pods	Zucchini squash
Bok Choy	Green beans	Parsley	Summer squash
Eggplant*	and **Okra***		

*These two vegetables have a gooey starch component that is especially good for lowering cholesterol. Slice up some eggplant, spray on a bit of olive oil and grill it. Cholesterol-lowering therapy never tasted so good!

Recipe: Grilled Eggplant

Wash a fresh eggplant, and slice into ½" thick slices, across the eggplant

Brush or spray with olive oil.

Grill over medium hot coals, turning every 3 – 4 minutes. Slices are cooked in about 8 to 10 minutes.

Season with balsamic vinegar, salt & pepper, tomato sauce or grated Parmesan cheese.

Some starches are especially rich in the fiber that lowers cholesterol.

Notice on the food list in the next page that black beans, kidney beans, and lentils are all listed there as starches. People often think, "Oh, rice and beans; rice is the starch, and beans are the protein item." The amount of protein in a half-cup of beans is 7 grams, about equal to a 1 oz. slice of turkey or cheese. Accompanying the 28 calories of protein is another 100 calories of carbohydrate. So while they offer a few more grams of protein per cup than most "starch" foods like corn and potatoes, you can still view kidney beans, split peas, lentils and chickpeas or humus as starches. The extra protein and fiber-content in beans makes them digest slowly, keeping blood sugar and insulin responses low as people digest them. They are the ultimate "low glycemic load" starch. Low glycemic load means slow digestion, and low blood sugar rise after eating.

STARCHES: High fiber starches are nourishing, and are good for weight control.

Black beans	Pinto beans	Chick peas	Potatoes	Plantain
Kidney beans	Lentils	Humus	Sweets potato	Corn
Pea beans	Pumpkin	Limas	Winter squash	Peas

GRAINS: Whole grains have more fiber than white ones. Try:

| Buckwheat | Oats/Cheerios | 100% Rye bread | Brown rice | Oat Bran |
| Quinoa | Corn tortillas | Barley | Millet | (Wheat) |

Notice, how wheat is here, but in parenthases: (Wheat). Wheat is a grain, and whole whole wheat is a possibility, but I am finding many people are more comfortable when they move away from eating wheat on a routine basis. So yes, whole wheat bread has more fiber, but there is an issue of whether it promotes some inflammation, which would raise the risk of having cholesterol stick to arteries, and raise the incidence of having extra calories turn to abdominal fat more readily.[253] I also find in my clinical practice, having people eat less wheat, even whole wheat, reduces their acid reflux.

Two Germans, Wolfganz Lutz, MS and Christian Allan, PhD., wrote a very interesting book called "*Life Without Bread*[254]", and have many positive case reports of how people look and feel better after having stopped eating wheat and many less grain foods in general. Their food plan is higher protein and lower carb as well, but particularly suggesting that people be wary of grains. I am not stressing the avoidance of all grain, but I am urging people to use other carbohydrate sources like fruits and legumes more often. I am also suggesting that people eat barley, brown rice, buckwheat, and quinoa more often, plus spelt and millet. Save the wheat for fun stuff like pizza or pasta pesto. Use 100% rye bread for sandwiches.

NUTS & SEEDS
Essential fats also matter to lowering cholesterol numbers and reducing risk of cardiovascular disease.[255] Cholesterol travels through the blood in protein-fat droplets called lipoproteins. These droplets hook up to lipoprotein receptors on cells: the first step in getting cholesterol to move from arteries on into cells. Next, a lipoprotein "lipase" grabs the droplet and levers it on into cells. The primary fuel to run the lever is an essential fat labeled GLA – gamma linolenic acid.[256] This is a fat found mostly in seeds, and in plants like Evening Primrose and Borage. The body can convert only a small amount of the fat in corn oil and vegetable oils—linoleic acid (LA) – into GLA, so direct sources in the diet are important. I often suggest that people with dry skin, and high cholesterol, take 2 Evening Primrose Oil pills per day, 1000 to 1300mg each, for 3 months, and then get their cholesterol checked.
Lowering Cholesterol and Heart Disease risk, cont. ...

Many times, people coming to me for cholesterol reduction advice will say,

*"I don't understand it, the longer I am on my low fat and
low cholesterol diet, the higher my cholesterol goes."*

I'll then say, "And tell me how dry your skin is."

Their eyes widen, and they reply,

"How did you know?" "My skin is incredibly dry. I have to use skin lotion all the time; and I hate it, in the winter, when the skin on the tips of my fingers cracks and hurts."

The tough fact is, people are too often told (erroneously) to avoid all fats, to lower their cholesterol and reuce their risk of heart disease. In the process they cut down on oils, and they certainly avoid seeds, which are known to be fatty. So they end up having a deficiency of GLA, which is the oil that is the moisture barrier in the skin, as well as the fuel to support the peripheral (around the edges of the body) cholesterol lipase lever I just mentioned.

In addition to a focus on the essential fat in seeds, many nuts still support lower cholesterol numbers. In most studies, almonds have some properties that lower cholesterol numbers.[257] Remember too, that nuts have many nutrients, like magnesium, that will help not only cholesterol numbers, but also help weight loss and blood sugar numbers in people with type 2 diabetes.[258] Walnuts also have added anti-inflammatory action on the cells lining arteries. [259]

Here is an example of a good clinical case, using fruits, probiotics, and essential fats to lower LDL cholesterol.

> Betty is a 61 year-old woman who came to see me, since she was hoping to avoid the Lipitor her doc wanted her to take. She was already eating a low cholesterol, low saturated fat diet. Her weight was normal. Her cholesterol was 301. Before you gasp, her HDL was 100. Her TG's were normal, and her LDL was 178. She represents a dilemma. Her Cholesterol to HDL ratio is less than 3.5 to 1, so in one respect, her tremendously high HDL offsets her high cholesterol. Someone else would say that the LDL must be lower, down to <159 no matter what. However, high cholesterol matters to pre-mature heart disease, but she is over 60 and doing well. She took a small beta-blocker pill; not for hypertension, but to prevent her heart from occasionally having a fast beat.
>
> In discussing her diet, she agreed that she could eat 3 fruits a day, instead of the one to two she currently consumed. She said that her stools sank in the toilet. She did not have dry skin, though she consumed few seeds, and her main oil for cooking was olive, not a source of GLA.

I encouraged her to take one probiotic pill a day until her poops floated, (it took 2 weeks,) and asked her to eat 3 fruits daily. Rather than consume sunflower and pumpkin seeds, which she didn't really care for, I suggested that she take 2 Oil of Evening Primrose pills a day, 1000 mg each, as a source of GLA. She would take these until she had her next cholesterol check. In 3 months she emailed me the results of her lipid check. It was nice news. Her Cholesterol was down a few points, but her LDL dropped 27 points, down to 163, and her HDL rose even higher, to 107 ! Her physician was happy with these numbers and she could skip the prescription Lipitor.

I still encouraged her to take 2 grams a day of fish oil, for the EPA/DHA to keep her arteries slippery, and to eat colorful foods, especially red grapes, so her cholesterol would not be oxidized, and cause inflammation in her arteries, and to take an antioxidant multivitamins with 100 iu of "natural" vitamin E each day.

The good cholesterol news inspired her to spend a little more time on her bicycle too, so now her heart attack risk would drop even lower.

The bottom line ... If you are over 60, and don't have heart disease, and don't want to be on a statin or other drug, your diet and exercise program are the most potent heart disease prevention therapy you can do, much more potent than taking some medicine. You and your doctor may feel more comfortable getting your cholesterol level down a bit, so do the following and see how your numbers play out.

1. Exercise 30 minutes per day, 5 times a week.
2. Eating the saturated fat of beef/meat twice a week is ok.
3. Eat the saturated fat of cheese, in 1 oz. servings, just every 2 or 3 days.
4. Eat fruit three times a day.
5. Eat 1 pound of vegetables a day.
6. Take one or two fish oil pills a day, to achieve 500-1000 mg intake of EPA/DHA, if not consuming fish 3 times a week.
7. Take two evening primrose oil pills per day, 1000 to 1300 mg each
8. Take a "probiotic" supplement often enough to get stools that generally float.
9. If HDL is low, take 2 grams per day NAC - N-acetylcysteine for 3 months.

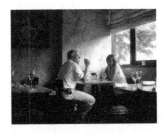

MANAGING HIGH TRIGLYCERIDES

High triglycerides (TG) means you have extra fat (grease) in your blood stream. If the numbers are above 700 for a while, you could develop an inflamed pancreas, known as pancreatitis. This can be deadly, because it can cause you to get infections and kidney failure.

Also, with that much grease in your blood, you feel tired. It is most likely the result of some medicine you are taking, (likely the combination of protease inhibitors added onto nucleosides like AZT, D4T, 3TC, FTC, etc.) but eating too much fat and sugar can also contribute to the problem. Here are some steps to take to reduce your triglycerides.

If your TG level is above 300, start doing something about the situation.

1. **Aerobic exercise** is a great treatment. A 45-60 min. power walk or a treadmill session is effective. Bicycling or roller blading for 45 minutes is good too. Try to do it all at one time though, a 30-minute walk twice a day isn't as effective. If 2 half-hour sessions is what you can manage though, that is very useful.

2. Lower the grease level in your diet. **Ease up on fatty foods** like ice cream, cheese, snack chips and French fries. Eat some good fiber foods, like more vegetables and fruits, and bran cereals. Olive oil is the best choice for cooking oil and salad dressing. Canola is ok, but doesn't have the anti-inflammation proterties that olive has.

3. Take **3 grams Fish Oils** each day. Also known as Omega 3 fatty acids, code letters EPA/DHA. These can be good for lowering inflammations too. DON'T take fish oils if you have low blood platelets. You might raise your risk of bleeding too easily. (Ask your expert HIV nutritionist about taking N-acetylcysteine (2 grams a day) to raise your platelets. Take this for a month or two. Ground flax seeds (1-2 Tblsp/day) or flax seed oil pills (2 gm/day) may be used instead of fish oils later on, but start with fish oils. By the way, ground flax seeds have a great nutty taste

4. Take **2 grams Evening Primrose oil** each day. This an omega-6 essential fat. It can help prevent heart disease, helping lipase (fat-clearing) activity. It can help it raise "good" HDL cholesterol levels too. It also solves the dry skin problems that people get when taking some protease inhibitors.

5. Take **1 gram L-Carnitine** each day for 2-3 months. This is crucial if you have TG's greater than 700. This improves the ability to burn fat. It can lower cytokine (stress hormone) levels as well. Carnitine comes in prescription form "Carnitor" too; ask your doctor about it if you find it helpful. You may hear about acetyl L-carnitine; it does not help burning fat as much, but it may be helpful for preventing or reversing neuropathy left over from taking 'd' drugs, like ddI, ddC ,and D4T. Carnitine and fish oils are helpful with Norvir-containing HAART, like with Aptivus.

The fibrate drugs like Lopid are only slightly useful. Ask your doctor about prescribing this only after your exercise and fish oil and L-carnitine supplement efforts aren't working well enough.

Selenium and antioxidants seem to reduce risk of pancreatitis. These should all be a part of your vitamin supplements when HIV+ anyway.

High triglycerides are sometimes a suggestion that your HAART drugs are increasing your blood sugar, and have you pointed in the diabetes direction. Again, if your sugars are creeping up, take the L-carnitine for 6-8 weeks.

You can reduce diabetes risk. Glucose is managed by insulin. Insulin works with glucose tolerance factor (GTF). GTF is composed of Glutathione, Niacin, & Chromium. Over time, you can expect your chromium levels to be low due to the nutrient malabsorption caused by HIV infection. Take 200 mcg chromium/day for 1 month. Niacin is part of the B-complex you are taking. Taking 2 gms NAC/day for a month, plus continuous 5 grams L-glutamine helps maintain good glutathione levels.

Insulin receptor status on muscles is a function of "in-shape" level of muscles, and repair status. Do some resistance-training exercise: this means weight lifting.

Alpha Lipoic Acid (200-600mg/day) can also help sugar pass through muscles better, and might reduce neuropathy risks thanks to its antioxidant effects on nerve cells. Alpha lipoic acid also helps keep glutathione levels higher.

Testosterone levels also impact sugar processing and storage in liver. Have your free testosterone levels checked if your sex urges are low, or if your TG's are high.

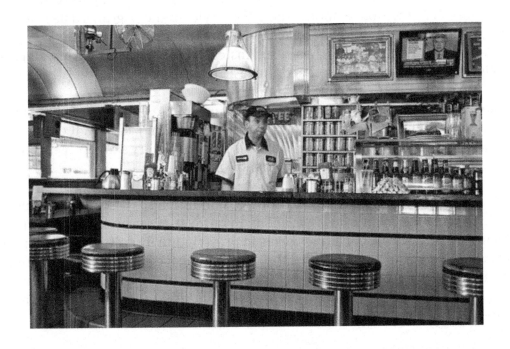

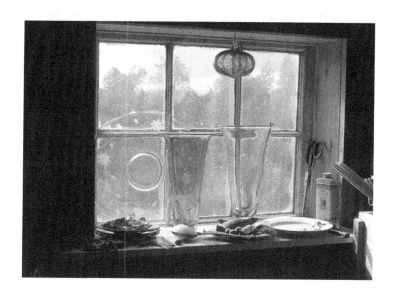

Quinoa Salad Recipe

Quinoa boils up like rice, simply add twice the water for the amount you cook.

1 cup quinoa, rinsed, and scant 2 cups water ... boil 12-15 minutes.

Now add some assortment of salad vegetables, to become 3-4 cups, all diced into ½ inch cubes when possible.

I recommend 1 red pepper, 1 green or yellow pepper, 2 4" pickling cukes (skin on)
1 small Vidalia onion or 6-8 scallions (tops and bottoms chopped)
When tomatoes are in season, and taste decent, add one.

For dressing, whisk together 1/3 cup freshly squeezed lemon juice and 2-4 Tablespoons of a tasty olive oil. Add in:

¾ cup finely chopped fresh cilantro or parsley.

Stir dressing over the salad, serve warm, or let chill in refrigerator for a few hours.

You can cook the quinoa ahead, and just chop veges and add to already chilled quinoa.

Quinoa provides carbohydrates, but it is a seed, not a grain, so no gluten issues.

New Information: An Extra Heart Disease Risk Found In HIV Infection

You have heard the risk factors for heart disease are conditions like age, high cholesterol, high blood pressure, smoking, etc. You can calculate your risk of having a heart attack, based on your numbers. A popular formula to use is the Framingham Risk Score (FRS).[260] [261] There are a number of web sites where you can calculate you risk of having heart trouble in the next 10 years. These formulas predict risk, based on the likelihood of "calcified plaque" found in arteries.

Meanwhile, something else is occuring in people with HIV infection. A less common "non-calcified plaque" seems to be accumulating. None of the usual predictor equations apply to its presence. Framingham Risk Score is not helpful. Significant arterial blockage can be happening in people at a younger age than expected, like early forties. A unique marker for immune activation and inflammation, soluble CD163, seems to be the risk factor, according to neuro-endocrine researcher Steve Grinspoon, MD.[262] He reports that this is a marker for "Innate Immune System" activity. He also points out that non-calcified plaque is less stable than calcified, and the risk of a piece breaking off and causing a heart attack is higher in this type of coronary artery disease. To quote his concern: *Development of non-calcified lesions related to persistent monocyte activation may predispose HIV-infected patients to plaque rupture and premature CAD.*

Is there any therapy that might reduce this risk pattern? Dr. Grinspoon wonders whether some of the immune activation is coming from the gut, as LPS? Lipopolysaccharide (LPS) is a sugar-fat molecule, remnants of gram-negative bacteria cell membranes, that gets through the gut wall and into the blood stream when the gut bacteria are not keeping intestinal cells in full repair. You may already have heard of "leaky gut." Even being on effective ART, the gut immune system is not operating at ideal level, so there is more LPS in the blood, suggesting more gut debris is enetering the blood stream and challenging the immune system.[263] Read more about gut eco system in "Taking Care of your Intestines" section of this book, page 91. I suspect that L-glutamine as gut repair material would be helpful. Soluble CD163 is a marker for innate immune activity, which suggests that Co-enzyme Q10 supplements may have some utility here too. There is an analogy in Type II diabetes, Co Q10 supplementation reduces inflammation in arteries.[264] Remember, less inflammation means less cholesterol will be sticking to arterial walls.

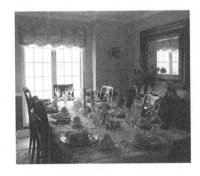

Hypertension:

As people age, they sort of expect to need blood pressure medications. Many people with hypertension end up on two or three medications to maintain control of their blood pressure. The side effects of pressure-lowering medicines include: fatigue, headaches, cough, swelling of hands or feet, muscle cramping, dizziness, lightheadedness, low potassium and impotence. The stress of chronic infection taxes blood pressure regulation nutrients in the body. In the area of blood pressure management, when I ask, "Is it aging, is it HIV, is it the meds," I seriously want people to focus on nutrition, so that management of blood pressure is simpler.

The science lesson: Fine muscles in the walls of arteries and veins contract and relax to maintain a certain amount of pressure in the vascular system. There are a number of hormone-like chemicals in the vascular system, that regulate relaxation and contraction of those vessel wall muscles. The kidneys have a role in fluid volume in the blood stream. As we age, the muscles and the cell walls of this vascular system may be a little less pliable. Organs become slower too. The assortment of chemicals that regulate fluid volume often operate with a little less precision as well.[265]

Usual nutrition advice for lowering blood pressure is reducing sodium level in the diet. The mineral sodium attracts water. Extra sodium in the blood and tissues brings in water, and the added volume in blood vessels raises pressure. It seems like there is sodium in everything: bread, pasta, milk, and cheese, let alone cold cuts, soups and catsup. People often get frustrated trying to avoid it, and abandon the sodium reduction effort. Truly avoiding sodium is difficult, and people just don't do real well with it.[266] Furthermore, the reward for being on a low sodium diet feels like a life of bland foods.

Interestingly, if the body were just better at pumping sodium back out of cells, then pressure drops back down. Researchers at The Brigham and Women's Hospital in Boston figured out that people consuming more of the minerals **Magnesium, Potassium,** and **Calcium** excrete sodium better, and blood pressure does stay lower, even for people who don't eat strictly low sodium diets.[267] They have a Web Site that details how to eat. What you'll notice, there, is that much of the dietary components are Cave Person food fundamentals: more fruits, more legumes, and many more greens. **See details of the D.A.S.H diet at www.dashdiet.org.**

An even more dynamic and focused intervention for lowering blood pressure naturally comes from some professors at the University of Vermont. In their book, called **The K+ Factor**, lead author, Richard Moore, PhD points out that the ratio of Potassium (symbol K+) to Sodium (symbol Na+) in milk, nature's first food, is 3:1. His research has shown that if someone eats a diet that has 3 parts K+ to 1 part Na+, then, it is quite hard to have an elevated blood pressure. [268]

A simple example: if you have a bowl of Cheerios, 160 mg sodium per cup, you have to offset that with 480 mg of potassium, which happens to be the amount in one banana.

Look in the tables below to see how the K Factor food plan would play out in a modern versus a Paleo era breakfast. See how you could concoct hypertension therapy for this meal. Notice, 2 slices of bread provide an average of 300-400 mg sodium, so you need 900 to 1200 mg K+ to offset the bread's Na+. A medium banana will provide the 500mg K+. A milk or yogurt is kind of a neutral: 375 mg K in a glass of milk, but 125 mg Na+. You still need to come up with 300 mg or so of potassium. An orange for a snack would do it.

Notice the mineral balance in a modern, grain-based breakfast, compared to the Paleolithic breakfast I am encouraging. The numbers are all in milligrams.

"Modern Food Plan Breakfast"

Food	Serving	Potassium	Sodium	Magnesium	Calcium
Whole wheat toast	2 slices	50	400	20	40
Smart Balance	2 teasp.	3	60	0	0
Orange juice, fresh	4 oz	236	1	12	11
Coffee	10 oz	145	6	9	6
½ & ½	2 Tblsp	39	12	3	32
Sugar	2 teasp	0	0	0	0
Totals		473	479	44	89

The K Factor here in modern breakfast is 0.987, a bit less than 1 : 1

Paleolithic Breakfast

Food	Volume	Potassium	Sodium	Magnesium	Calcium
Salmon	3 oz/wt	369	49	28	38
Banana	1 large	487	1	37	7
Almonds	15 avg	127	0	48	48
Tea	10 oz	110	9	9	0
Milk	1 oz.	43	13	3	36
Honey	2 teasp	7	1	0	1
Totals		1143	73	125	130

The K Factor here in an old world breakfast is 15.6 … almost a 16 : 1 ratio …

If you at all wonder how well the K factor works, here's some proof. Six months into the initial publicity tour promoting the book, its success was becoming apparent. Pharmaceutical company pressure forced MacMillan publishing to stop the tour. The authors discuss this at their website: http://www.minconf-forests.net/drug-books/richard-moore-md-phd-drugs-are-not-the-answer-for-high-blood-pressure!

Blood sugar levels also play a role in blood pressure level.

Another nutrition connection to blood pressure to appreciate is carbohydrate calorie loads. You have heard of the hormone insulin. When people eat fruits and starches, as those foods digest, blood sugar levels rise. Insulin tells cells around the body to open up and absorb sugar from the blood. However, Insulin has *build fat*, and *retain sodium* and *make hungry* messages too. Think about a modern breakfast. By the time you add up the amount of carbohydrates from a typical breakfast: 2 slices of toast, plus large banana and 4 oz. milk, you end of with 61 grams of carbs: (30 toast, 25 banana, 6 milk). This is 244 carb calories. Insulin responds to rise in blood sugar, and ends up telling the hormone aldosterone, in the kidney, to retain sodium.[269] In other words, blood pressure can go up when the size of carbohydrate servings are substantial or excessive. If breakfast were a caveman-era blend, of protein-fruit-nuts, BP will stay lower. If you make breakfast a whey protein and banana smoothie, plus a handful of almonds instead, there is less insulin released. Having low sodium-low fat cottage cheese, small banana, and 2 tablespoons of raw, unsalted sunflower seeds can also produce an impressive K:Na ratio (37:1) and maintain a low insulin response.

(See Diabetes section, pages 108) for more information on insulin activity.)

The Heart As a Pump

Are you over 50 and looking for a little more energy? Think about providing your heart with a little more fuel. The heart pumps 5.6 liters of blood though the body in about 20 seconds. Each day, blood travels 12,000 miles and the heart beats 10,000 times!

You may remember from some old biology courses that fat and sugar are converted to the energy form called ATP in the Krebs cycle. ATP is the energy currency for muscles. This all happens in the mitochondria, oven-like units inside all the cells in the body, including cardiac cells. There is a vitamin-like substance called Co-enzyme Q10 inside the mitochondria that completes the ATP production process. I call Co Q10 the velvet lining inside the walls of the mitochondria

The quality of the heart's pumping action is measured as *ejection fractions*. Having lower Co Q10 levels in the heart can mean less available fuel, so less capacity for strong ejections.[270] Not long after age 20, production of Co-enzyme Q10 starts going down in the liver and in muscles.[271] By age 50, Co Q10 levels can be inadequate for ideal heart function.

As we age, Co Q10 levels can be less than optimal in our heart and other cells. We get Co Q10 in the protein foods we eat: fish, chicken, eggs and meats. This isn't quite enough to meet our needs. Usually, the liver converts the Co Q7, Co Q8 and Co Q9 found in fruits and vegetable to Co Q10 to complete the supply for the heart's needs. After age 50, the liver simply doesn't do this so well. Supplementation may be needed.[272] Also, statin drugs, the ones everyone takes to lower cholesterol, reduce Co Q10 production in the liver.[273] So age plus medicines compromise the ability of the liver to supply heart tissue with adequate Co Q10. You want to appreciate what Co Q10 does for you and see if you feel better taking it.

Karl Folkers, a researcher at The University of Texas, was the man who first described the chemical structure of Coenzyme Q10, in the late 1950's. He conducted a number of trials, using Coenzyme supplementation in many cardiac cases. The routine result was that ejection fractions improved. Another consistent effect was that people reduced the amount of blood pressure medication they needed to take.[274]

You remember, I mentioned Dr. Folkers before? Co-enzyme Q10 is fuel for Natural Killer cells, which play a continuous role in managing HIV infection. Here is the point in BP management. If the immune system is soaking up the limited supply of Co Q10, then there is less around for the heart. You end up on more BP meds, and risk more side effects, when just taking more of the nutrient Co Q10 is the better solution.

The Heart and the Innate Immune system are competing for a diminishing supply of Co Enzyme Q10 in people over 50. The result: lower Natural Killer cell activity, and rising blood pressure.

Most people taking Co Q10 find that they have a bit more energy in their day-to-day life. There is no risk to health in taking it. I will not interfere with prescription medicines with one exception. If you are taking several blood pressure medicines, after a month or two of taking Co Q10, you will likely have to lower your dose of BP medicine, or you could end up hypotensive: having low pressure and being dizzy.

Again, you can take the BP meds, and ignore the nutrient issue, but that neglects an important part of your immune system capacity. Remarkably low levels of Co Q10 are found in people with breast, lung and pancreatic cancer. Low Co Q10 levels are predictive of poor prognosis in the cancer called melanoma.[275] Its use, along with some other antioxidants, has helped people with breast cancer have better remission rates when on a breast cancer chemotherapy treatment program.[276] A new study coming out in the journal Blood describes how the chemotherapy drug Rituxan (Rituximab) works by locking on to tumor cells in such a way that NK cells come in for a 60% better kill rate.[277]

Heart Failure

Heart failure is the diminished capacity of the heart to pump enough blood for the body's needs. The heart is a muscle, and as it ages, it can become weaker. One consequence is less ability to pump fluids around the body. Picture the image: blood is pulled to the feet by gravity, but cardiac contractions must push the blood up from the feet and back through veins, to the heart. If the pump is sluggish, fluid pools in the ankles and lower legs. The medical answer is to use a drug like Lasix, «a fluid pill» that keeps people a little drier, and there is less fluid to leak into the extremities. Anyone with the swollen ankles of heart failure knows it is down-right annoying and painful. Swollen tissue hurts. Imagine the swelling of bee stings around both ankles, all day and night. Anything that could be done to prevent this is worth knowing about. Here is an abstract from a congestive heart failure journal: [278]

Title: **Nutritional assessment in heart failure patients**.
Journal: Congest Heat Fail. 2011; 17(4):199-203
Authors: Lee JH, Jarreau T, Prasad A, Lavie C, O'Keefe J, Ventura H.
Source: John Ochsner Heart and Vascular Institute, Ochsner Clinical School, The University of Queensland School of Medicine, New Orleans, LA, USA.

Abstract (**bold letters** added by me, Charlie Smigelski, RD)

Heart failure (HF) is a growing epidemic worldwide with a particularly large presence in the United States. Nutritional assessment and supplementation is an area that can be studied to potentially improve the outcomes of these chronically ill patients. There have been many studies reporting the effect of various nutrients on HF patients, often with mixed results. Amino acids such as taurine, which is involved in calcium exchange, have been reported to improve heart function. **Coenzyme Q10**, a key component in the electron transport chain, is vital for energy production. **L-carnitine**, an amino acid derivative, is responsible for transport of fatty acids into the mitochondria along with modulating glucose metabolism. **Thiamine** and the **other B vitamins**, which serve as vital cofactors, can often be deficient in HF patients. **Omega-3 fatty acid** supplementation has been demonstrated to benefit HF patients potentially through anti-arrhythmic and anti-inflammatory mechanisms. **Vitamin D** supplementation can potentially benefit HF patients by way of modulating the renin-angiotensin system, smooth muscle proliferation, inflammation, and calcium homeostasis. Although supplementation of all of the above nutrients has the potential to benefit patients with HF, more studies are needed to solidify these recommendations.   © 2011 Wiley Periodicals, Inc.

Notice all the nutrients accented in **bold** letters are ones that are helping manage various aspects of HIV infection. Being sure your levels are in optimum supply could help you either dodge or treat other medical issues, like heart failure.

Studies of nutritional care in heart failure have usually intervened with just a single nutrient. If heart cells are low in 4 to5 items, clearly a single agent wont help much.

There have been just a few small combo studies, and the results look good. The author **JeeJeebhoy**, in the abstract below, is a giant in the world of sophisticated nutritional research studies. [279]

Title: **Conditioned nutritional requirements: therapeutic relevance to heart failure.**
Journal: Herz. 2002; 27(2):174-8.
Authors: Sole MJ, Jeejeebhoy KN.
Source: University of Toronto, Toronto, Canada.

Abstract
BACKGROUND:
The advent of disease, genetic predisposition or certain drug therapies may significantly alter the nutritional demands of specific organs. Several specific metabolic deficiencies have been found in the failing myocardium: (1) a reduction in **L-carnitine, coenzyme Q10, creatine,** and **thiamine--nutrient cofactors** important for myocardial energy production; (2) a relative deficiency of **taurine**, an amino acid integral to intracellular calcium homeostasis; (3) increased myocardial oxidative stress and a reduction of antioxidant defenses. Deficiencies of carnitine or taurine alone are well documented to result in dilated cardiomyopathy in animals and humans. Each of these deficiencies is amenable to restoration through dietary supplementation. A variety of nutrients have been investigated as single therapeutic agents in pharmacologic fashion, but there has been no broad-based approach to nutritional supplementation in congestive heart failure to correct this complex of metabolic abnormalities.
METHOD AND RESULTS:
We have demonstrated deficiencies in carnitine, taurine and coenzyme Q10 in cardiomyopathic hamster hearts during the late stage of the cardiomyopathy. In another study, we randomized placebo diet against a supplement containing taurine, coenzyme Q10, carnitine, thiamine, creatine, vitamin E, vitamin C, and selenium to cardiomyopathic hamsters during the late stages of the disease. Supplementation for 3 months markedly improved myocyte sarcomeric structure, developed pressure, +dp/dt, and -dp/dt. We also documented **carnitine, taurine and coenzyme Q10** in biopsies taken from human failing hearts, the levels correlating with ventricular function. A double-blind, randomized, placebo-controlled trial of a supplement containing these nutrients, given for 30 days, restored myocardial levels and resulted in a significant decrease in left ventricular end-diastolic volume.

CONCLUSION: These experiments suggest that a comprehensive restoration of adequate myocyte nutrition may be important to any therapeutic strategy designed to benefit patients suffering from congestive heart failure. Future studies in this area are of clinical importance.

Compound Nutritional Support For Impaired Hearts

What people need to appreciate is that heart failure is not just about the heart. It is a systemic condition, characterized by much inflammation and inadequate repair materials. Repair materials in short supply can be materials like vitamins B2 and B6.[280] Lower levels of sulfur compounds like cysteine are also an element of inadequate repair in the heart.[281] At the same time, the clean up system is struggling: circulation is compromised, so toxins build up, and so do stray electrons. There is more «cytokine» (chemical messenger) activity, which generally leads to a feeling of fatigue. Cytokine messages also can contribute to insulin resistance. There can be a Catch-22 situation, as elevated blood sugars also trigger inflammation and vascular dysfunction.

Of course, it is smart nutrition to the rescue. As you have been already reading, any time food and vitamins can reduce inflammation, people generally feel better and their bodies function better. Science is sometimes looking at glutathione peroxidase levels (a key antioxidant enzyme) in people with heart failure. You already know, this is a major antioxidant enzyme for the whole body. Its competence depends on adequate protein and antioxidant nutrients like vit C, vit E, selenium and cysteine intake. This is a reminder that your Paleo diet and smart vitamin support are fundamental. It is also a reminder that says if you're feeling sluggish from heart failure, look to nutritional supplements to improve your ejection fractions and energy.

You have already read about B-complex vitamins, Vit D and Omega 3 fats in the previous pages here. So you are likely to be eating them in your food, and getting some extra amounts in your better-than-average multivitamin supplement. Taking Co-enzyme Q10 is the newer item here.

So, heart failure is simply the heart not pumping enough. It can be from age, corrosion or other damage. It can also be from not having enough fuel to pump as vigorously as would be nice. If you are feeling like your heart needs some more ooomph, to manage fluids in your ankles better, give Coenzyme Q10 supplementation a try. See what kind of energy improvement you may experience too. Take 100 mg, twice a day for 4 to 6 weeks.

Important, inform your physician that you want to take Co Q10 supplements for energy. Again, there is no toxicity to the Co Q10. The issue is that when it starts working for you, you may need to reduce the amount of heart regulation medicine you are taking. See the anecdote (next page) ...

With heart failure, a person's energy keeps dropping. Added nutritional support generally means people feel added energy, which contributes a lot to quality of life.

With poor blood circulation, cells lining the intestine are also at risk for not functioning properly. The gut's barrier function is compromised, and «debris» (science words: endotoxin or lipopolysaccharide) from inside the intestines, gets into systemic circulation, and causes inflamamtion. As part of helping reduce all-over inflammation in the body of someone with heart failure, (CHF), think of how the gut is doing. (see Gut Ecosystem, next section) for more info on this.

Here is an interesing heart failure case.

An 80-year-old man was sent to see me when he was told his elevations in blood sugar were nearing the diabetic level. He was already taking medicines for blood pressure and heart failure and atrial fibrillation; he was taking Lipitor for cholesterol. He hoped to not start even more medicines for diabetes now, so wanted to manage his blood sugars with better diet. Of course I outlined a caveman style diet for him, including a cottage cheese and banana and walnuts breakfast. Lunch remained a simple tuna or turkey sandwich, since he was still working, and that is what the local deli near his office could provide. Supper became a baked potato or sweet potato almost nightly; I wanted him to have the potassium, to push the sodium out of system. I also urged salmon a few days a week, so the fish oils would keep the electrical part of his heart healthy and lots of vegetables, for the potassium. His heart was weak, and his ankles often swelled with fluid. He was taking furosemide (Lasix), a fluid pill, to reduce the pooled water in his lower legs.

Remember now, his age, and his being on a statin drug meant his Co Q10 levels were going to be at risk for being inadequate.

I asked him to take a better antioxidant multivitamin that included B-complex, plus 100 mg Magnesium, and 100 mcg selenium. I also started him on 100 mg Co-enzyme Q10, twice a day, for 8 weeks, then taper to once a day for maintenance. His heart began pumping better, thanks to the Co Q10. After 3 weeks, he no longer needed the Lasix fluid pill. At 6 weeks, his doctor also lowered his blood pressure medicine doses too.

I have had this same experience with dozens of patients. Within a few weeks of taking Co Q10, blood pressure is naturally lower, and BP medicines are reduced. Again, I mention Coenzyme Q10 because of its importance as Natural Killer Cell fuel, and its use as an antioxidant for arteries.

I want to quote Dr. Folkers here.[282]

Title: Usefulness of coenzyme Q10 in clinical cardiology: a long-term study.
Authors: Folkers K et al. Journal: Molecular Aspects of Medicine, 1994.
15 Supplement, pages 165-75.

"Before treatment with CoQ10, most patients were taking from one to five cardiac medications. During this study, overall medication requirements dropped considerably: 43% stopped between one and three drugs."

This is tremendous results! People end up on less medication, so have fewer side effects. Plus, people feel an improvement in their basic energy level.

The man's blood sugars normalized. It was probably a combination of elements that helped the sugars get better. Better eating kept blood sugar lower in general. A better vitamin helps insulin talk to muscle insulin receptors more effectivly. Co Q10 made for better heart function so better blood flow helps clear out metabolic waste in the body, which lowers cytokines that can cause insulin resistance. Less vascular inflammation helps reverse insulin resistence too.

It is a Catch 22 with heart failure, people feel week, and exercise less, but more fitness activity would lead to better "conditioning" and improve wellbeing. Co-enzyme Q10 is good for raising energy levels in people with heart disease.

Nutrition can help break the cycle: low energy prevents the exercise that would improve energy and conditioning. All kinds of athletes use the amino acid **L-glutamine**, to improve muscle repair after workouts, and improve performance during training. You already know it is a good idea to be taking omega **3 EPA/DHA** for general health and brain function. A study at Columbia-Presbytarian Hospital in New York showed that use of both glutamine and EPA/DHA together improved exercise capacity in people with CHF (congestive heart failure). Again, get some professional help to try this for your self.[283] L-carnitine , at a dose of 2 grams per day has improved muscle action in heart failure trials too.[284]

Conclusion: when feeling sluggish and frustrated because of heart failure, find a dietitian that can inform you of careful intervention with a few key nutrients: Coenzyme Q10, antioxidant multivitamin, L-glutamine, omega 3 fats and L-carnitine. Discover how these supplements will improve your quality of life.

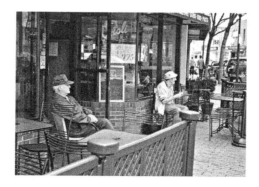

Intestinal Health

There is an old Greek adage, credited to Hippocrates: *All disease starts in the gut.* This was certainly quite an insight, as the gut ecosystem is critical territory in regular life, but even more so for people with HIV.

The stomach and intestines are a complex metabolic system. The GI – gastrointestinal -- system is a tube, approximately forty feet long, running through the body. People swallow food, and it's on its way to the toilet, unless it digests down to small enough molecular particles that can pass across the cell walls of the gut on into the blood stream. Think of the skin of your cheeks: the cheeks at either end of your body even! The skin rounds the corner and becomes the lining of the tube, either down the throat or up the butt. It is still "skin", though it now becomes very specialized in its function. It must let selected food particles into the body, but then a little farther down the tube, it has to hold back some nasty shit. Quite a sophisticated set of cells, eh? Clearly, you want that skin / gut cell lining seriously well nourished, so it can perform its job perfectly, especially its barrier function.

Many people experience their intestinal system not working well. Irritable Bowel Syndrome (IBS), (sometimes called Spastic Colon) affects about 15% of the US population. Research conducted by The National Institute of Health, revealed that more than 60 million people suffer with heartburn associated with acid reflux disease once a month; and 25 million people are daily sufferers of the disorder. National Health and Nutrition Examination Survey statistics suggest that 10% of the population have the problem of constant constipation. The incidence of GI dysfunction increases with age.[285] Sometimes it is unclear if the problems are an issue of aging physiology, or side effects to other treatments. For example, many medicines have a constipating side effect.[286] Anti-anxiety pills like Amitriptyline, pain pills like Oxycodone and Tramadol, plus Buprenorphine and Methadone come to mind. Colitis, which is extra immune and nervous system activity in the large instetine, is a common problem. Think about it; in a group of older people, hanging around chatting, the conversation frequently turns to GI difficulties. Remember the Aunties in "Arsenic and Old Lace?" One complained of *dyspepsia*, and everyone knew what she meant.

Science Lesson
View the 40' long tube called the GI track as its own ecology system. There are several hundred species of bacteria and microbes living there. Among them are some beneficial species. These are labeled "probiotics", since they are the opposite of antibiotics. The GI system has more nerve receptors for serotonin than does the brain. There are many immune cells produced in the G.A.L.T. = Gut Associate Lymph Tissue. Nutrients manufactured by friendly bacteria in the gut (gut flora) are important to the health of cells lining the colon, and to cells in other locations, like the lungs. The status of this eco system matters a lot to gut comfort and function.

An View of the Gut Ecosystem : cross section of intestines

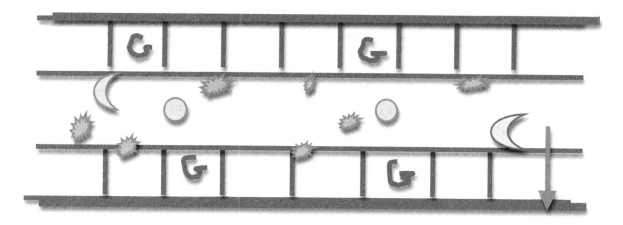

 = probiotic species, like lactobacillis and bifidobacter

 = pectin-rich fruits like apples, pears and bananas

 = G.A.L.T ... gut-associate lymph tissue (immune cells)

 = food passes through intestine cells to enter the blood stream

Diet is the major force in gut health. Foods and their fibers determine what microbes flourish in the gut ecosystem. The indigestible fibers in vegetables, fruits, grains and legumes, are food for the gut flora. A diet rich in fruit fibers, like pectin, plus the beta glucan fibers found in oats and legumes, (kidney beans, lentils and chick peas), supports a bigger population of desirable microbes.[287] These beneficial microbes will tend to suppress the growth of undesirable gut bugs, like yeasts and staph bacteria. The right or wrong set of gut flora also impact tendency to weight gain and to develop diabetes.[288] [289] You have already read about how good gut bacteria also make small fat particles that help reduce cholesterol production in the liver. The small fat particles are also important repair fuel for cells lining the colon. In general, people with a good gut flora population in their GI ecosystem, will have stools that float, when they have a bowel movement. I tell people "fruit-fiber-floaters" when it comes to their gut health. If you are not eating your 3 fruit servings a day, then it is hard to declare yourself nourished. At the same time, I'd be worried that your good gut flora are at risk for starving, and I'd worry about colon cells not being in their best state of repair. This compromises the ability of the colon to act as a tight barrier, and to hold back some bad news bugs from seeping into the body. I remind people, they are really just one flush away from the local sewer system. Clearly gut flora population matters. As I said a minute ago, there are pills available that people can take, to install a good set of gut bugs. The pills are "probiotics".

Many items people ingest can disrupt the GI ecosystem. The artificial sweetener sucralose seems to reduce good flora population.[290] Consuming too much alcohol is disruptive too.[291] Acid blocker drugs (like omeprezole, "the purple pill Nexium") can shift flora pattern to higher population of E coli (Escherichia coli) and yeast (Candida albicans) species.[292] This is not good. Older people taking these acid reduction meds experience higher rates of pneumonia, presumably from the change in gut flora pattern as well. [293]

Having a comfortable bowel movement most days of the week is important.

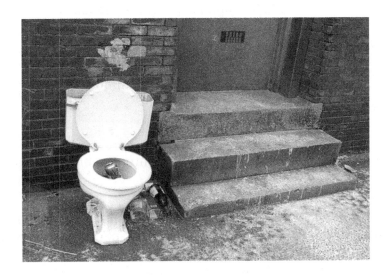

avoid constipation

Building A Better Bowel Movement

- Eating enough **fruit fiber** is the first step toward assuring comfortable bowel movements. Fruit pulp nurtures the useful gut flora population. For this, be sure you are eating fruit three times a day.
    - A banana a day is a good idea. No, they are not constipating or fattening. They do offer great fiber, which solves both constipation and diarrhea. A medium banana is 100 calories, not too fattening. Have a handful of nuts or seeds with any fruit to slow its digestion, if blood sugar is a concern.
    - Also have an apple or pear. Applesauce and canned pears work too.
    - A serving of berries is a good idea too, as both GI system and brain food.

- With constipation or diarrhea problems, take **a probiotic** that is a blend of Lactobacilli and Bifidobacter species.[294] A capsule that delivers 5 billion "colony forming units" is a good place to start. I have good clinical results with a product called *JarroDophilus EPS.* (I have no financial interest in this company.) It is simply a product that works for people, at a reasonable price. Take a probiotic for a week or two. Once stools float, you can take it less often, or stop it altogether, until sinkers happen, or until some gut symptoms return. Occasionally I recommend the probiotic *Culturelle*. It has good antibiotic properties, so when someone has "small bowel bacterial overgrowth" as part of their finicky colon, I treat them with *Culturelle,* two pills a day for 4 weeks.

- The amino acid **L-glutamine**, sold in powder form, is repair material for cells lining the intestines. When sensing that you want better repair function in your GI system, try ½ teaspoon of L-glutamine, taken once or twice a day. See how it makes you feel. Read an excellent book by Judy Shabert, MD, MPH, RD called *Glutamine, The Ultimate Nutrient*, published by Avery[295], if you want more details on it. Just put the ½ teaspoon, 2.5 grams dose, L-glutamine powder on your tongue and wash it down with a gulp of water. It is tasteless. It is often energizing. Warning, you may also feel a bigger zoom from your coffee and other caffeinated beverages when taking L-glutamine. One precaution: pregnant women should not take glutamine. It is unstudied there. Read more about L-glutamine in the next section, GERD remedy. Handy to know, in cases where I worry about some gut infection, I use Glutamine at higher doses: 1 Tablespoon 2 or 3 times a day for a week or 10 days. This worked well in the old days of crypto- and microsporidia infections.

Help With Acid Reflux and GERD

Acid reflux can happen for any age people. The treatment is usually drugs to limit acid release in the stomach. I already mentioned that proton pump inhibitors and H2 agonists meds can disrupt gut flora. It would be nice to see if the acid regulation system could be re-set, to work properly. The following plan has helped my patients, young and old. Give it a try. It costs you about $30 for your two-week experiment.

Reflux is fluid flowing in reverse, up from the stomach, into the lower part of the esophagus. When stomach acid washes up there with the flow, this is "acid reflux". Why this happens is not well understood. In part, the valve at the top of the stomach does not close enough, and acidic fluids leak upward. So far, though, the medical goal is just to stop the acid part of the backwash, so that no damage happens. Acid eroding the cells of the lower esophagus for too long can cause scarring and cancer: (Barrett's Esophagus) so people go on prescription acid blocker drugs, like Omeprazole/Nexium. Just an FYI, long term use of those drugs can sometimes lower vitamin B12 levels in the body[296], and increase risk of osteoporosis.[297] Acid blockers mess up the balance of friendly flora in the gut, increasing the incidence of community acquired pneumonias in older people. If using these medicines long term, try to keep the dose as low as possible.

Usually the system that regulates stomach acid production is in the cells in the wall of the stomach. Stomach acid is really the body's disinfectant system. In the olden days, foraging in the forest, food wasn't as clean as what we eat now; it seems that the body developed stomach acid as a way to kill off germs and bacteria as we ate. When stomach acid is done disinfecting, acid production is supposed to stop. Some researchers feel that if production isn't quite high enough, the system keeps on churning out more acid. An analogy: the leaky toilet tank that keeps running, because it never hits the high water mark and never shuts itself off. A popular home remedy that many people find useful for acid reflux is consuming 1 Tablespoon of apple cider vinegar at the end of a meal, to contribute a little more acid. I have no clinical experience with this, but feel like it is worth passing on. Many Internet reports must be worth something. If you try the vinegar, don't mix it with bicarbonate. Just use a little water.

With acid reflux, it seems that there is something else provoking more acid production and secretion. There is some speculation that further down the intestines, some cells are also telling the system to generate acid. One idea is that the acid/alkaline level in the lower part of the small intestine has something to do with controlling acid emission. While stomach contents are very acid (a pH of 2), intestine contents are supposed to be very alkaline (a pH of 9), for the final phase of digestion. The bicarbonate coming out of the pancreas raises the pH of the gut to make it alkaline. If the pH does not rise high enough in the intestines, maybe stomach acid keeps pouring out. A pH at 8 or so is the reason for Kaletra diarrhea. Look into Pertzye.com if you are having protesase-induced diarrhea.

Another idea: wheat proteins are the culprits. In earlier times, wheat was a diploid, 2-chromosome protein. The current model being grown is hexaploid, 6 chromosomes, for better crop yield and resistance to disease. This modern wheat can sometimes be very irritating to intestine cells; many people are finding out that avoiding wheat keeps their gut system happier. [298] The structural changes the cells seem to make in response to the chronic distress is that the cells generate acid secreting signals. Now one of the possible interventions is to stop eating wheat for a while, so this system fades away. Avoiding wheat is not the same as avoiding all gluten, a protein found in wheat, rye, oats and barley. After a few weeks of no gut cell wheat hassle, it is ok to eat some wheat again, but not on a daily basis.

Gut Rehab - Food and Nutrition Supplements for Gut Ecology to Reduce Reflux

The nutrition concept here is to get the whole gut ecosystem in its best shape, so that the pancreas is working at its best, and cells lining the gut are repairing well.

Step 1 for having a good gut ecosystem, then, is eating a lot of water-soluble fibers. Start with eating 3-4 servings of fruit per day. Ideally among those fruit encounters, you eat one banana, or one apple or one pear each day. These fruits have the most pectin. The fruits can be fresh, frozen, canned or dried, anything to get the fiber.

Another useful fiber to try to eat every few days is oat bran. It cooks up like cream of wheat. It's a decent cereal. It is great as a mid-morning snack. Use Cheerios or oatmeal on other days.

Add a tablespoon of ground flax to applesauce or oat bran cereal. It tastes nutty. The fiber in flax nurtures good gut flora.

Step 2 is taking some Lactobacillis pills, sometimes called "probiotics". A brand I recommend: Jarro-Dophilus EPS pills, 2 per day. Another good one is Culturelle.

Step 3 is taking some L-glutamine each day. Glutamine is gut cell repair fuel. It is also immune cell fuel. It helps buff up the intestinal ecosystem in a variety of ways.

1 Tablespoon of L-glutamine powder provides 10 grams. You want to take <u>10 grams, twice a day</u>, for about 2 weeks. Just dissolve the glutamine in an ounce of cool water or juice and drink it down. Don't mix it in anything hot. Take it 5 minutes before breakfast and supper.

If you are a coffee drinker, or consuming a lot of caffeine in sodas, you may notice that you will get more of a caffeine buzz when taking glutamine. Pregnant women should not take Glutamine, as it is an immune system booster. If you have Crohn's disease or rheumatoid arthritis or other immune related diseases, glutamine is actually good to take. In auto-immune cases though, start the L-glutamine gradually, like 1 teaspoon a day, for 5 days, and increase by 1 teaspoon every 5 days. Note, 3 teaspoons equal 1 Tablepsoon.

After two weeks avoiding wheat, and of taking probiotics and glutamine, you could try reducing your Nexium, Zantac or Pepsid, etc. and see how you do.

Go to www.vitaminshoppe.com to buy the JarroDophilus EPS pills. They also have good prices on L-glutamine. You'll need the 400 gram container of glutamine for the

2 – 3 week trial. The Vitamin Shoppe brand of L-glutamine is Body Tech. That is a reputable product at a good price.

Again, a Paleolithic Food Plan, avoiding wheat, would look like this. Adjust portion sizes to meet your caloric and appetite needs. Here's approximately 1800 calories.

		Calories
B:	protein: 2 oz. turkey, 3 T. whey protein powder or 2 eggs, cooked	100
	fruit: a sm. banana, 3/4 cup fresh or canned fruit	80
	nuts: 1 Tblsp. peanut butter or handful of nuts or seeds	100
	dairy: 6 oz. no-fat yogurt or 8 oz. skim milk	80
	bev: black coffee, regular or green tea	
Sn:	starch: 1 c. oatmeal or 1.5 c. Cheerios	150.
	or fruit: a small box of raisins or 1 cup applesauce	
	bev.: 4 oz. glass of skim milk	40
L:	protein: 3 oz. salmon, sardines, turkey or chicken	150
	starch: 1/2 cup kidney beans or lentils or 1 cup peas or potato	150
	veges: 2 lg. carrots, or a tomato and a green pepper	60
Sn:	dairy: 8 oz. skim milk, or 1 cup yogurt	80
Sn:	nuts: 1 handful (2 T.) walnuts, almonds, cashews	100
	fruit: a lg. peach, 3/4 c. pineapple chunks, or 1 apple	75
D:	protein: 4 oz. broiled fish, poultry, or lean meat	200
	starch: 1 cup green peas, corn, limas, baked potato	150
	veges: 1-2 cups broccoli, cauliflower, spinach, carrots, etc.	80
	oil: 1 Tblsp nuts, 2 tsp. Smart Balance or 1 tsp. olive oil	45
Sn:	fruit: a big orange or apple, or 2 plums or a kiwi	100
	dairy: 10 oz. skim milk or 1 cup no-fat yogurt	100
	Total calories:	1840

The maintenance plan to keep acid regulation going well is different for each person. Some people take just 1 probiotic once a week and 1 teaspoon of L-glutamine every 3-4 days. Others need the supplements a bit more often. They usually have a wheat food treat, like a slice of pizza, a muffin or some pasta just once every 3 or 4 days.

HIV, HCV, The Gut, And On-going Immune Activation

There are a lot of immune cells in the gut. The gut lining is a highly sophisticated eco system. Think about it; there are millions of "germs" living in your intestines, rubbing up against the cell wall, and somehow your gut is not excessively inflamed. Meanwhile, the system can jump on invading bugs when they happen in food poisoning. It is the GALT, gut-associated lymph system, that challenges unwanted germs like salmonella. Understanding how the resident array of good and bad gut bugs manages immune response is an emerging field of medical study.

In HIV infection, the gut is the site of much activity. HIV lands in the gut lymph early on in the infection process, depleting T cell numbers. This affects whole body T cell immune response.[299] Drop in T cell numbers in the gut is correlated with collagen deposit scarring.[300] The reduction in gut mucosal immune capacity compromises the gut cell wall as competent barrier, and something called microbial translocation occurs. This means the gut wall, as a barrier against bacteria in the gut is less competent. Ongoing leaky gut can be a reason for poor T cell recovery after starting meds.[301] Researchers are looking at LPS. (lipopolysaccharide) levels as a way of sensing leaky gut status and degree of ongoing immune activation from this area of the body.[302]

I am describing the gut T cell situation in detail for several reasons. Ongoing inflammation in the body is added work for the immune system. Inflammation is a risk factor for gene damage and cancer development. Higher LPS numbers from the gut represent a risk factor to Non-Hodgkin Lymphoma.[303] A lower CD4 cells count also is a medical risk, as you already know.[304]

Remember, a while back, I was talking about CD163 levels and risk of non-calcified cholesterol and chance of premature heart disease. There is not a lot of research data describing gut nutrient status and supplements and CD163. We do know a few things about L-glutamine and preservation of crucial gut monocyte and macrophage activity in infections.[305] We know that L-glutamine supplements help reduce pro inflammatory cytokine production in test tube models of gut cell metbolism.[306] We know there are bursts of inflammatory NF-kB and TNF-a cytokines when not maintaining good glutamine levels.[307] Healthy gut cells that get challenged with the irritation of some LPS are much less stressed when supplemented with L-glutamine.[308] Again, let me clarify, less stressed means they send out less distress signals that are going to alter whole body metabolism, including fat and sugar processing, and immune cell competence at fighting even the common cold.

I am using some connoisseurship here to strongly urge people to take 5 grams per day L-glutamine, and 1 probiotic pill most days, at 5 Billion or more Colony Forming Units a day, just to keep the gut system in its best possible state of repair. I can't show you an HIV study yet about the assured benefit. This treatment will cost you about $10 a month. You are spending the $10 to hedge your bets to reduce on-going immune activation and clogged arteries. Remember, in the heart section, I was talking about non-calcified cholesterol as a risk factor for clogged arteries? Dr. Grinspoon is wondering to what extent LPS and disturbed gut health may be triggering more CD163 expression. Again, I am advocating support of gut cell integrity as a precaution against this cholesterol plaque issue. In the meantime, the materials still have benefit to your basic wellbeing and your regular cholesterol levels too. I add an informative abstract here, to point out the area where this protection will play out. I placed the conclusion in **Bold** letters.

AIDS. 2012 Apr 24;26(7):843-53. doi: 10.1097/QAD.0b013e328351f756.

HIV infection induces age-related changes to monocytes and innate immune activation in young men that persist despite combination antiretroviral therapy.

Hearps AC, Maisa A, Cheng WJ, Angelovich TA, Lichtfuss GF, Palmer CS, Landay AL, Jaworowski A, Crowe SM.

Source

Centre for Virology, Burnet Institute, Melbourne, Australia. annah@burnet.edu.au

Abstract

OBJECTIVES:
To compare the impact of HIV infection and healthy ageing on monocyte phenotype and function and determine whether age-related changes induced by HIV are reversed in antiretroviral treated individuals.

DESIGN:
A cross sectional study of monocyte ageing markers in viremic and virologically suppressed HIV-positive males aged 45 years or less and age-matched and elderly (≥65 years) HIV-uninfected individuals.

METHODS:
Age-related changes to monocyte phenotype and function were measured in whole blood assays ex vivo on both CD14(++)CD16(-) (CD14(+)) and CD14(variable)CD16(+) (CD16(+)) subsets. Plasma markers relevant to innate immune activation were measured by ELISA.

RESULTS:
Monocytes from young viremic HIV-positive males resemble those from elderly controls, and show increased expression of CD11b ($P < 0.0001$ on CD14(+) and CD16(+)subsets) and decreased expression of CD62L and CD115 ($P = 0.04$ and 0.001, respectively, on CD14(+) monocytes) when compared with young uninfected controls. These changes were also present in young virologically suppressed HIV-positive males. Innate immune activation markers neopterin, soluble CD163 and CXCL10 were elevated in both young viremic ($P < 0.0001$ for all) and virologically suppressed ($P = 0.0005, 0.003$ and 0.002, respectively) HIV-positive males with levels in suppressed individuals resembling those observed in elderly controls. Like the elderly, CD14(+) monocytes from young HIV-positive males exhibited impaired phagocytic function ($P = 0.007$) and telomere-shortening ($P = 0.03$) as compared with young uninfected controls.

CONCLUSION:
HIV infection induces changes to monocyte phenotype and function in young HIV-positive males that mimic those observed in elderly uninfected individuals, suggesting HIV may accelerate age-related changes to monocytes. Importantly, these defects persist in virologically suppressed HIV-positive individuals.

PMID: 22313961 [PubMed - indexed for MEDLINE]

The Gut Ecosystem and Better T Cell Counts

Having higher CD4 count numbers always feels psychologically better, at least for getting out of the 200 to 300 range and up into the 500's. Again, let me just discuss gut ecology and immune response and T cell counts. There is the issue of the aging immune system and something called "dysregulation". It is not just that things are sluggish; it is that chemical regulation signals lack their previous precision. There is a lapse into a pro-inflammatory state.[309] What does this mean? Think of it as a slight "itis" condition, almost low-grade fever in the region. Since 75% of T cells are manufactured in gut lymph tissue (GALT), this region needs to be supported the best you can. As mentioned before, probiotics and prebiotics (the food fibers like pectin that support probiotic health) can reduce excess inflammation in the area.[310] Proof of concept was reported at CROI, 2012, where *Culturelle*, a probiotic available at drug stores across America, improved gut Tcell count recovery in an animal model of SIV infection. This study has now just been written up in the *Journal of Clinical Investigation*.[311] Remember, cytokines (chemical messengers) like IL_1, Il_2, $TNFa$ and NFK_b rise in response to inflammation, ie free radical stress. In the long run, my concern is that oxidative stress, chronic inflammation, and cancer are closely linked.[312] In the shorter run, cytokine expression shifts metabolism in support of the immune and repair cell activity. Peripheral fat cells receive a continuous "release fatty acids" message. This raises fat content of the blood, which then triggers TNFa to generate insulin resistance, so as to keep blood sugar levels a bit higher, again as lymphocyte fuel. In a person who is ageing, or in someone with much extra body fat, this continuous sugar release into the blood will appear as maturity-onset diabetes. This is not your grandmother's diabetes, however. Diabetes drugs will not seem to have their usual efficacy either, as the situation is not an insulin receptor defect. It is cytokine messaging, and possible glutathione deficiency. [Note: the persistent cytokine messaging is part of the lipoatrophy of lipodystrophy.] This was all triggered by inflammation that started in the GI system.

The concept I want to accent is that modest support of gastrointestinal surface cells (enterocytes and coloncytes) and gut lymph cells is worth some attention, to reduce long run complications of subtle inflammation over time.

Taking L-glutamine at 4 – 5 grams per day, and some intermittent use of probiotics, is a good idea for reducing the inflammation that could increase risk of cancer, diabetes and heart disease.

Bone Health, Osteoporosis, Risk of Fractures.

Osteoporosis is high on the list of American women's health concerns as they age. Bone scans are a routine part of preventative medical care for post-menopausal women. Surgeon general's statistics indicate that 12 million people in America have osteoporosis, and 40 million have lower bone density to some degree.[313] The statistic that perhaps 20% of the people who have a hip fracture are dead in 12 months is chilling as well. As you know from your own life experiences, there is a vast range of health status among people 60, 70 or 80 years old. Some people at age 80 are out walking daily, while some 60 year olds are significantly impeded with arthritis, excess weight, diabetes, and heart conditions. Bone and muscle health together matter a lot.

In a certain way, it is the concept of vigor (strength and vitality) versus frailty (thinness and weakness) that is most operative, when assessing risk for fractures.[314] In an interesting Montreal study of 241 people, average age 75.4 years old, death rates after a hip fracture were higher in the people less than 70 years old, and lowest for people older than 80.[315] This raises the question, "Were the younger people actually more frail?" If it takes until you are 80 to fall and fracture something, you were likely in good shape for a long time. An Australian study points out that fracture rates start out higher in women, but catch up for men in their 80's.[316] Just so you know, nutrition can play a dynamic role in reducing complications and speeding recovery after bone repair surgery. An 8 oz. drink with 254 calories and 20 grams of protein, consumed once a day, shortened convalescence from 40 to 24 days in one hip fracture study. Complications to recovery, even 6 months later, were only 40% (versus 74%) in the nutritionally supplemented people too.[317]

So you have a bone scan, and hear that your bones are thinner than the standard 18 year old. **The situation is not so dire**. Again, I defer to *Overdosed America*, where Dr. Abramson questions why we are compared to the body parts of an 18 year old? As for how much to worry about osteoporosis, he reveals some interesting statistics in the Fossamax Study that got the drug approved by the FDA, for osteoporosis therapy.

Eight thousand --8,000—women, ages 55 and older, enrolled to get either active drug or placebo. In the course of 4.2 years, **95.5%** of 4, 000 women on placebo remained fracture-free. On Fossamax, the number of fracture-free women rose to only **95.8%** of 4,000.[318] Do you notice? The incidence of fractures is low to begin with, and the actual benefit occurs to **just three-tenths of one percent** (0.3 %) taking the drug over 4 years. Would you take a drug where you knew that just 1 person in 81 benefits in the course of 4.2 years? Would you ask about the side effects, like death of the jawbone – osteonecrosis of the jaw – causing your lower teeth to loosen and wobble? Recent analyses points out it also increases some atypical fractures and recommends just 3-5 years therapy at most.[319]

What I am most concerned about is that a focus on the (low utility) drug distracts people from actions that can be far more useful in fracture prevention and improving bone health. There are a number of nutritional and fitness moves associated with better bone health and true lower fracture incidence.

*The true health concept is: it is not so much about bone strength.
It is really about preventing the falls that result in fractures.*

The Key Elements For Preventing Fractured Bones

- **Toned muscles**: People whose muscles that have lost size and strength are more prone to falls. Eating enough protein is key to maintaining muscle volume. Doing resistance exercises, which means lifting weights or using exercise machines, maintains or even builds strength.

- **Tuned up proprioceptors**: Little sensors in the joints tell you what your arms and legs are doing: feeling muscle length and tone, and what angle joints are at. You don't watch your legs and feet as you walk, you look forward and inherently know how far out you have placed your foot as you take steps. Your proprioceptors (little sensors in joints) are letting your brain know what's going on in your limbs. You could eat with your eyes closed, and get the fork to your mouth, thanks to the same sensors. Proprioceptors can lose their sensitivity from lack of movement. It's like a muscle: use it or lose it. Routine fitness activity keeps proprioceptors tuned up; lack of activity leads to poor function and, for instance, less stability walking. Nursing home programs that have people doing just 10 minutes a day of muscle activity, like calisthenics, walking, stepping, or stretching, see a major reduction in falls and fractures. People, in modern life can end up quite sedentary, where they miss their "daily walk" or exercise bike activity for 4 to 5 days. Even this is enough for people to experience a reduction in leg coordination.

- Being **well-nourished** matters to bone strength. Get blood tests, be sure your **vitamin D levels are $\geq$ 50 nmol/L ($\geq$30 ng/ml)**. Adequate calcium and **magnesium** in the diet matter too, as you know now. The **D.A.S.H. diet**, that emphasizes more Ca++, Mg++, and K+ keeps bones stronger, too.

Knowing the exact amount of calcium, vitamin D and other nutrients to eat, to prevent or reverse osteoporosis is difficult. The DRI (Dietary Reference Intake) for vit D for seniors age 51 to 70 years, is 600 iu/day and for Elderly[320], over 70, is 800 iu/day. The recommended amounts for calcium are 1,000mg for men under 70, 1200 mg for women that age, and 1200 mg calcium for everyone over 70.[321] But ....

Osteoporosis and fracture rates are the highest in countries with the most milk and calcium intake. An example: in Bejing, women are consuming little milk/dairy, and average about 587 mg calcium intake per day.[322] Chinese women have some of the lowest age-related fracture rates in the world. [323] With urbanization, though, the rates are doubling, and then some, for both men and women. [324] This would suggest something about lower physical activity as a bone fracture risk factor. Interestingly, better bone density in another study of Chinese women, is correlated to fish and fruit consumption! [325] I would speculate that the fish are helping vit D levels, and the fruit is nourishing the GI system, so there may be less inflammation in the body. [326] Just as a point of comparison, in Japan, calcium intake averages 400 – 500 mg a day, coming from small fish with bones, soy products and vegetables. Osteoporosis rates are about 8% of the population, similar to the US numbers. However, fracture rates are less than half what they are in the US. [327] So along comes more discussion of whether milk/dairy is the place for assuring good calcium intake, and will that really help increase bone strength and reduce fracture risk. I would like to put in a word for feeling like fitness level may be most important for staying well, and having good bones.

Dairy intake may be of questionable usefulness. Interestingly, Harvard Medical School and Harvard School of Public Health offer their own version of "My Plate" for teaching healthy eating,[328] and it does not contain the small round glass of milk symbol that is part of the US Government / USDA My Plate nutrition advice program.[329] I have an impression that vitamin D and trace minerals like magnesium are under-appreciated issues in the thin bones arena. The inflammation factor does not get enough attention either. Of course the practical food advice to cover all of these pitfalls is here in this book.

If your bones are thin, and sometimes hurt, and you want to truly re-calcify them, look into the products by the **Algaecal company: www.algaecal.com** . Their bone remodeling data is the most impressive I have seen. In a way, calcium from algae mimics the calcium from leaves that we got in the olden days. The Algaecal people generated good bone remodeling with 540 – 720 mg per day added calcium, depending on diet to supply 700mg, the US women's average. The Algaecal plan also includes a supplemental mineral pill, which includes strontium, boron, vitamin K2 and other trace elements crucial to bone development. People with years or decades of HIV-related gut malfunction could likely really need these extra trace minerals.

There is some discussion about taking too much calcium in pill form. One Australian study detected more heart attacks in women taking calcium at 500mg per day, or more.[330][331] One study should not change all of clinical suggestions. I do suspect that an extra 500 mg a day is a sufficient boost to enhance dietary intake.

Remember, there is an important distinction: in studies looking at 77,000 women, yes, more calcium, vit D, and other minerals make stronger bones, but this did not translate into reducing fracture rates. [332][333] The bottom line: bone mineral level is not such a strong player in fractures. Falling is the problem. That's about muscles and strength and co-ordination then.

HIV Diease and Bones ... cont.

Thinning bones is a developing concern in HIV care. A look at a few hundred HIV+ men in New York showed bone thinning at more than twice the rate of some matching HIV-neg guys. People who used heroin, who had an AIDS diagnosis, and who have Hep C co-infection had more bone loss in this study. [334]

Many events can account for why this happens. Infection means there is more inflammation in the body. Inflammation reduces the ability to maintain full calcium levels in the bones. Many people have gone through a period of lower testosterone. This hormone matters to bone strength in both men and women. A paper published by the New England Research Institute in 2012, estimated the 20-year incidence of osteoporotic bone fracture due to testosterone deficiency in American men, age range 45-74, to be 600,000 cases, at a public health cost of billions of dollars.[335] A while back, there was an HIV treatment interruption study that had people cycle off their HAART when their T cells rose, as a way to reduce exposure to the toxicity of meds. The study was halted early, because people who went off treatment got sicker, including more heart attacks. Inflammation due to more viral growth when not on meds was the likely reason that people didn't do so well.[336] One other bit of information from that study is that people experienced much slower bone loss when off treatment drugs, despite the inflammation,.[337] Over the course of a year, there was even evidence of bone re-mineralization for those not on meds.[338]

Let me emphasize, medical people call the loss of minerals "bone disease". How much this clinically matters is still unknown. Yes, bones are not looking like people are 18 years old. Does this really translate into more fractures? Little research results are available yet. One Danish group says yes, higher rates of fracture are happening, and taking meds is part of the risk.[339] This paper spans the time period from 1995 to 2009. An Australian paper, from just 1998 to 2009 says meds are not an issue. Low CD4 count, anti-epilepsy therapy, and use of corticosteroids (drugs like Prednisone) were the risk factors.[340] As you would imagine, the toxicity of HAART has changed radically over that time period. It is hard to draw conclusions from this limited data.

Taking Care Of Bones While We Wait For More Data.

We know that bones are losing minerals early on in HIV infection, even before starting meds.[341] We know that vitamin D levels are low in the general population and that includes positive people, and especially dark-skinned people.[342] We know that thinner bones—osteoporosis—are not the primary risk factor for fractures. The real issue is muscle strength and conditioning, plus good diet. Remember the discussion of sarcopenia – muscle loss with aging – back when I discussed adequate protein in the diet, page 16.

Bone Wellness Summary.

Eat a diet that has many caveman elements: fruits, vegetables, fish and essential fats. We know that whey protein (from cow milk) stimulates osteoblasts (bone-building cells),[343] so enjoy Whey protein at breakfast often.[344] Know your vitamin D levels. Taking calcium and vit D supplements for a defined period of time can help rebuild bone.[345] Again, I would take Algaecal plus the strontium-boron-magnesium-copper blend trace mineral supplement along with this calcium source if really needing to rebuild bone. It appears to have the best data on bone improvement. (www.Algaecal.com)[346] As I pointed out before, the real risk factor for fracture is lack of fitness. So besides thinking about bone quality, think about your exercise and fitness level. Have some leg muscles and keep them toned.

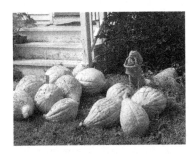

ELEVATED BLOOD SUGAR, PRE-DIABETES AND DIABETES

Nutrition and Metabolic Systems

A brief story ... I was hanging out at a local vitamin shop the other day, with my The Nutritionist is IN sign, on a table near the entrance. People come in, see my sign and me, and ask questions. This helps me keep in touch with what is on the public's mind in the area of nutrition, and I enjoy the chatting with the customers, many of whom are terrifically well read, thanks in part to Internet information.

A couple, appearing to be in their late 60's, came up to me and the woman was asking if the 1000mcg Biotin pills she was holding would help her grow thicker hair. (1,000 mcg is 3.3 X the RDA) I replied that I knew people sometimes grew less hair in a biotin deficiency, but I didn't think that added Biotin would produce more hair. She mentioned that she was already taking B-complex vitamins, as part of her supplement regime. (These frequently have a Biotin component, so she was unlikely to be deficient.) I suggested that she look into the product called BioSil ... basically silicon pills, that many people do find beneficial for growing stronger nails and thicker hair. She had not heard of this, so was going to do more reading before she bought it.

As she mentioned that she was taking many supplements, I asked if what was using included L-glutamine, Co-enzyme Q10 and anti-oxidant multi-vitamins, and she said,

"No". I suggested that this basic array would support more general repair in her whole body's systems. I urged that she first take this baseline support, and then, in 3 or 4 months, see what might be needed for specific parts, like hair and nails. I also asked is she was having a protein food item at breakfast. She answered, "No."

The woman's question points out the mind-set of many people when it comes to nutrition. Their approach is much like Western medicine, "What is the symptom, what pill will treat it?" Nutrition is seldom this simple. Nutrition is milieu therapy: you want to be sure all the essential ingredients are present, in correct proportions, for systems to run well.

Here's an example of how nutritional care is more complex. Since calcium is the major component of bones, at one time people just worried about having plenty of it to be sure bones grew strong. Then the effects of vitamin D on bone calcification became known, so adding vit D supplements became standard. There is a small magnesium component to bone structure, so some forward thinking companies add magnesium to the supplement mix, the same is true for boron and vitamin K2 now. Meanwhile, what people are not looking at is whether the body feels like directing all these resources to bones. If there is an excess of stray electrons, (free radicals), coursing through the body, all the food and supplements won't get to bones, other systems will get priority. Osteoporosis will still happen, even in a resource-rich setting. Good diet and smart supplements won't work if the milieu is not right.
As you just read in the previous pages, the gut is an ecosystem. Having it in good shape involves multiple items: a variety of food fiber, good bacteria, and sometimes certain extra amino acids. Wanting other body parts to work well too, like hair or nails, can also involve a mixture of repair materials. For a nutrition solution, don't just think about a body part and the pill to fix it. Think about broad-spectrum metabolic support.

For a nutrition solution, don't just think about a body part and the pill to fix it. Think about broad-spectrum metabolic support.

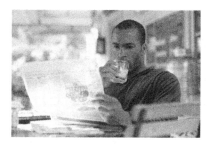

Be informed about the complexity of nutritional healing.

Carbohydrate & sugar processing ... Insulin resistance ... Diabetes

In the course of aging, many processing and repair systems in the body function a bit more slowly. Included in the decline is the handling of carbohydrate calories, as managed by the insulin system.[347] Most people, even without some family history of blood sugar issues, will have some decline in insulin signal and receptor function as they age. Added to this could be the shifts in metabolism caused by inflammation of arthritis, or lung conditions, intestinal glitches or chronic viral infection. A decline in muscle tone with age will also impede sugar processing. Mitochondrial damage, from age, medications, or illness will also hamper glucose clearance. The result can be that it all plays out with blood sugar levels remaining a little higher after meals.

Science Lesson
The body has a system for maintaining a steady supply of blood sugar to the brain, and distributing extra sugar from meals onto other body parts. After you eat pasta, potatoes, apples, peas, etc. digestion breaks down their carbohydrate calories to glucose, the sugar molecule – $C_6H_{12}O_6$ – you heard about in high school. So the glucose travels in the blood stream until the pancreas puts out insulin to process it. The hormone insulin essentially tells the cells that are next to arteries to open up and let the sugar molecules move on in. Insulin keeps doors open for about 20-30 minutes. Sugar moves into muscles for a while, but then the doors close, leaving a decent amount of sugar in the blood, to feed the brain. In juvenile (Type 1) diabetes, there is suddenly no insulin to do this job. The word *diabetes* actually means "sugar trapped in the blood". There is also "adult onset (Type 2) diabetes", where there is generally plenty of insulin, but the "move sugar" message is being ignored, or actually "resisted. "Insulin resistance" is the term describing this. "Impaired glucose tolerance" is another term for the slower movement of sugar out of the blood after meals. While "diabetes" describes the condition where sugar is trapped in the blood and not moving into cells, for Type 2 diabetes (DM2) "impaired sugar clearance" is a better term. In some situations, there is supposed to be some more sugar left in the blood, like in cases of infection, where immune cells may need the fuel. So "trapped" doesn't apply.

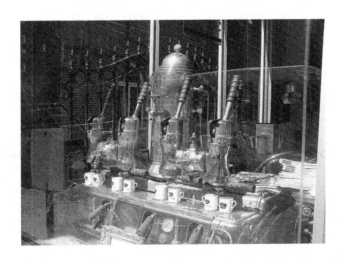

Insulin Action On Cells

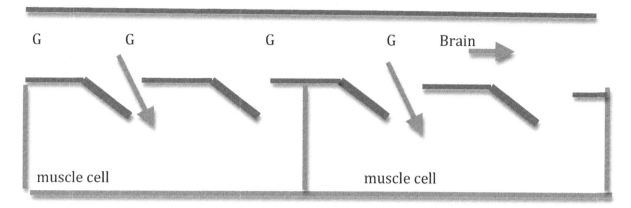

G = Glucose ▬▬▬ The cell door that Insulin tells to open, and let sugar in.
➡ sugar moving ... either to the brain, or into muscles and other cells.

The body provides a steady level of blood glucose to the brain at all times. When people eat, and blood sugar levels are higher, then insulin comes along and opens some doors to muscle and other cells, and diverts the extra sugar into the cells, so they can have fuel to function. Technically, it is not a door, but a protein structure – the GLUT4 enzyme – that insulin tells to escort sugar from blood on into cells. Think of it as a lock and key system. The insulin key is inserted into the keyhole/receptor, unlocking the door to allow sugar to enter the cells.

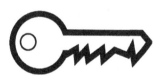 

Insulin / Key   Receptor / Keyhole

In thinking about moving sugar around, think about the status of the key and the keyholes. Is there enough insulin? What about the keyholes? Are there enough, are they corroded, or is something blocking their opening? For people getting adult-onset diabetes, it is not about lack of insulin. It is about the receptor functionality. Insulin sluggishness or absolute insulin resistance can be provoked by many cell system and events.

When people with HIV and HCV develop blood sugar problems, it is time to make a close examination of their metabolic status at that current moment. The major underlying mechanism for elevated sugar is an insulin receptor dysfunction, likely a response to inflammation.[348] There are fuel-processing systems to consider as well. Many times the body may actually want sugar to not be absorbed into some cells, so that it can be readily used in others. The body may also want to preferentially burn fat when there is too much of it someplace. Example, when clogged with too much fat, the liver tries to keep sugar out of its cells, so it "resists" the insulin message that is telling it to absorb the glucose. Insulin receptor activity is influenced by many body systems.

When there is too much insulin resistance, over some period of time, a diagnosis of diabetes happens. Type 2 diabetes (DM2) shows up as higher sugar in the blood of a person generally after age 50 or 60, though some late 40's diagnoses occur too. A recent phenominon is obese 16 years olds are also getting the DM2 diagnosis.

When people hear that they have diabetes, the language and culture of the medical industrial establishment gives them the impression that they now and forever will have this "disease". The vibe is that they will need medicine to manage this problem, for the rest of their life!" I want to raise a red flag about this, however.

I want people to step back and take another view: a view separate from the business model of the diabetes diagnosis. Yes, you have extra sugar in your blood, which is not good, and you have some amount of insulin resistance. Now, please think, "Why this insulin resistance now?" Are there some parts of me that are stressed and need repair or is my metabolism shifting due to some condition?

**Initially, Type 2 diabetes is a *symptom*;
the <u>problem</u> is usually excess inflammation!**

Most important: if you have Type 2 diabetes, don't feel as though you have now begun some automatic progression of continuously more complicated medical regimens. Take a step back and do a whole body assessment. What needs repair?

Read through the checklist on the next few pages, to see which body systems may be contributing to insulin resistance, and could use some attention.

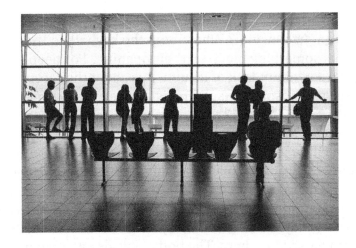

The Conditions That Generate Insulin Resistance
Or Diabetes That Are Alterable Are:

Change What You Are Eating
My observation is that in the last 10 years or so, as soon as someone has any high blood sugar lab results, they are put on the drug Metformin. In earlier times, a decade or four ago, a doctor may ask the person to try to control their blood sugar with diet. Food patterns can be changed. I point this all out, because I like to save medications for when they are really needed. In the famous *Diabetes Prevention Trial*, there was focus on diet and exercise, versus Metformin treatment in people with slightly elevated blood sugars. The results were that smarter food choices and more fitness activity reduced sugar levels much better than taking the drug Metformin did. Also, blood pressure and cholesterol medicine pill requirements dropped for the whole next decade, even.[349]

Are you really eating well?
Food changes, alone, can make a difference in glucose metabolism. Eating more red meat, cheese, refined grains, and less wine is the food pattern associated with developing diabetes,[350] A move to more caveman cuisine is a start toward better health. Over-eating both fat and carbohydrate calories causes inflammation.[351] Again, inflammation causes poor insulin function. Simply eating less food can begin to reverse diabetes. Making specific food changes also lowers blood sugars. A key element is the extra oxidative stress (inflammation) caused by too much of the wrong kinds of fat in the diet. Antioxidant vitamins, and a change to using just olive oil as your cooking oil, can improve sugar processing.[352] Remember, a supper of grilled shrimp or scallops, basted in garlic-infused olive oil, served on top of a spinach salad is a diabetes reversal prescription.

Shrimp, grilled with garlic olive oil, served over a spinach salad is diabetes therapy.

Some foods and some nutrient imbalances can cause inflammation. An excess of high fructose corn syrup[353] in the diet, or excess fructose in the setting of insufficient magnesium,[354] and even an imbalance in the ratio of calcium to magnesium can all impair the ability of insulin to clear sugar from the blood[355]. Magnesium is a tricky nutrient in aging and blood sugar issues. An older intestinal system may not absorb magnesium well. Insulin resistance causes disruption in magnesium flow. Low magnesium at the cell level causes more insulin resistance.[356] Remember to be eating magnesium foods daily, and get 100 mg or more in your vitamins. Better diet to remove these stumbling blocks is easy, still. You know the solution: turkey sausage, applesauce, and smoked almonds for breakfast.

You read about magnesium, back on page 40.
Can you name 5 good magnesium-rich foods now?

Exercise and Fitness

Remember, being "out of shape" also known as "under-exercised" is three times as risky for your health as having a high cholesterol count. The condition of muscles also matters to insulin response and glucose clearance. What can you imagine doing to start getting some conditioning going? Walking 30 minutes has significant positive health benefits. I urge people to do some upper-body muscle toning activity too. Most sports stores sell big rubber bands with handles and a wall chart of exercises to use them for. You can be "pumping rubber" while watching television. Whether carrying excess weight or not, starting an exercise program can reverse insulin resistance.[357]

Are You At A Healthy Weight?

Even if you are carrying just an extra 10-15 lbs of body weight, do something to reduce it. Obviously, diet and exercise are the smart place to begin. Where you carry your extra pounds, has added meaning. Weight in the belly area, versus spread out all over the body, means more risk of blood sugar and blood fat problems.[358] This is the apple shape (fat above the waist) versus pear shape (below the waist) description that you may have heard about. I add the waist:hip ratio info here, because I hope that you'll really work on improving your numbers if you are at risk.

Calculate your Waist: Hip ratio.

Measure your waist at the belly button, in inches.
Measure your hips at the widest part across your butt, in inches

Do the math: ___ waist inches divided by hips inches = ___ W/H ratio;
or use an on-line calculator if you want, Google gets you to a few.

Men	Women	Category	(Risk of health
0.95 or below	0.80 or below	Low Risk	complications, like
0.96 to 1.0	0.81 to 0.85	Moderate Risk	diabetes, hypertension
1.0+	0.85+	High Risk	heart disease.)

A higher Waist:Hip ratio is an indication that inflammation levels are higher than they should be. Trying to lose belly fat is harder than usual weight reduction. I urge people to use some supplemental support. Supplements include a better-than-average antioxidant vitamin as I have been mentioning all along. Also, take 3-4 grams per day fish oils.[359] Frequently, belly fat causes the blood fats called "triglycerides" to be high. If concerned about triglycerides, then add 1 gram per day of either the amino acid called L-carnitine or the one called acetyl L-carnitine[360] for a few months. The supplements help liver cells burn fat better. After 2 or 3 months, as weight loss is progressing, I just depend on dietary protein to supply the L-carnitine. Just an FYI, it is L-carnitine that provides the "gamey" taste in meats like lamb; mutton (adult sheep) is the best dietary source. That's not a popular food these days, in the USA anyway. Beef has more L-carnitine than chicken, pork or fish does too. Another reason why I advocate eating grass-fed red meat once a week or so. Grass fed lamb is available in many stores, like Trader Joes. Sleep-deprived people also tend to gain fat in the lower abdomen. Be well-rested.

Body Mass Index is another calculation. It is weight, divided by height-squared. Again, go on-line and Google BMI calculator. There are many options. BMI greater than 30 means obesity. The obese label certainly carries a lot of emotion with it. I mention the term here just for a point of science, or medical fact. Significant excess fat creates conditions that impair glucose processing. Again, it is all about inflammation. Fat cells, especially those in the belly area send out distress signals. One distress signal generates insulin resistance. Think about it. You are a fat cell, you don't want to get any bigger; next time someone is trying to deliver excess sugars to you to store as fat, you're going to resist the message. It is also about the physics. Fat is taking up space, blocking insulin's access to receptors on cell surfaces.

Extra fat in the gut area often accompanies a condition called "fatty liver." A liver that is choking on excess fat will also send out a signal to resist the efforts of insulin to send in more sugar. [361] As mentioned above, fewer calories, fish oils and carnitine are the best remedial strategy for unclogging a fatty liver.

I promote authentic nutrition first, and diabetes medicines second. Weight gain is a common side effect of diabetes treatment. Extra fat weight gets in the way of good blood sugar control. Why does the weight gain happen? The medicines are forcing sugar into liver and fat cells, making them store fat they didn't want to have in the first place. In the case of the thiazolidinedione drugs, (Avandia and Actos) this therapy seems to increase risk of heart attacks,[362] and some cancers. [363] I feel very comfortable claiming that a few extra caveman nutrients are the best initial intervention in blood sugar problems. A few extra vitamins, plus fish oils and L-carnitine don't give people heart disease or cancer! The Linus Pauling Institue has some excellent information of how good L-carnitine is in treating people with heart failure, kidney failure, peripheral vascular disease, diabetes, and HIV.[364]

Nutrients That Are Crucial To Insulin Working Well
Lets talk about some more nutrients that may be deficient and that is why people develop blood sugar problems. Vitamin D is high on the list. Something about having decent vit D levels keeps sugar moving better.[365] You seriously need to know where your vit D levels are for many reasons, anyhow. (page 41). Chromium, a trace mineral, is crucial to carbohydrate metabolism. Many health food stores and nutrition books will recommend it for diabetes care. I am conservative on this one. You can get 100 to 200 micrograms of Chromium per day in a smart vitamin supplement, and that is a fine dose.[366] Higher doses over time could disrupt the absorption of other trace minerals and cause deficiencies that would be hard to detect.

Nutrients that are part of cell construction are subtle modulators of glucose metabolism. A deficiency is hard to detect or describe. For example, EPA/DHA omega 3 oils are also an item that could be low, and this will effect insulin action, but there is no easy way to detect this. All cell membranes are made up of the fat molecules we eat. A cell can survive on corn oil or lard in its structure, but it will function better when it has a certain amount of EPA/DHA fat in its structure. In this case, the insulin message is more effective when there are EPA/DHA molecules in the muscle and liver cell membranes.[367] Certain amino acids present in muscle cell surface proteins also help carbohydrate processing. L-glutamine is a key player here. It exerts its influence in many metabolic realms for glucose management. One is that glutamine helps muscles be in their optimum state of repair, so that insulin receptors are in good shape too.[368] Glutamine also has a role in improving insulin signaling.[369] The amino acid Arginine helps glucose tolerance, as well.[370] [371] Glutamine helps support better Arginine levels in the body, so I don't recommend taking extra Arginine. L-glutamine accomplishes a lot on its own.

L-glutamine is extra special
I find the amino acid L-glutamine a very useful supplement for many patients, especially those with blood sugar problems. People with diabetes or insulin resistance frequently have mood problems. The hard part to figure out is which came first, the mood problem or the diabetes.[372] It can be the worry over food management and blood sugar testing, and the experience of hypoglycemic events that wears people down. It can be lifestyle elements, like less exercise or less nutritious eating in depression that cause the insulin resistance.

When in doubt, I first vote biology, then psychology. Common to both diabetes and depression is a higher than usual amount of inflammation in the neuro-endocrine systems, plus a failure of the immune system to bat clean up enough.[373] Deeper analysis of brain metabolism in people with diabetes and depression is the discovery that their brains are low in L-glutamine.[374] Well, studies of people who are receiving L-glutamine as part of bone marrow transplants treatment for cancer show improvement in mood.[375] Again, it can be a simple one teaspoon dose of L-glutamine powder, (4.5 grams), each morning. The only people who should not take extra Glutamine are people on a protein-restricted diet due to their advanced liver or kidney disease. Pregnant women should not take glutamine either, but then, that is not a likely event for the primary audience of this book. One warning, glutamine does often make people feel the effects of caffeine more intensely. Careful of the coffee buzz when you are taking some glutamine.

Check Hormones
Hormones also have a big influence on sugar metabolism. As part of reversing sugar processing problems, you might consider knowing what your hormone levels are.

For men, a low testosterone can mean more blood sugar issues.[376] The extreme example of low testosterone: men on hormone suppressive therapy as part of their prostate cancer treatment are at much higher risk for diabetes.[377] Men may want to know their "total" and "free" testosterone levels, when working on reversing insulin resistance. If testosterone levels are low, my first vote is to look at some lifestyle issues, like excess alcohol intake[378] that might be the cause. Getting adequate sleep matters too.[379] If considering treatment, look into Eastern medicine treatments first, like Tong Ren (see page 133) and acupuncture. There are prescription testosterone gels to try as well. I prefer getting the body's own systems working naturally if possible. Testim® is the gel that seems to be most recommended by the sharp endocrine docs around Boston. Steve Grinspoon, MD, at Mass. General Hospital does wonderful investigations of hormones and lipodystrophy in people with HIV. He describes how various medicines affect abdominal body fat accumulation. More importantly, he has shown that testosterone replacement therapy reduces gut fat, improves lean body mass, and reverses insulin resistance problems.[380] Men with prostate health issues, like elevated PSA, are not to go on testosterone therapy. For anyone interested, though, Dr. Abe Morgentaler in Boston is researching whether this is actually the best advice.[381]

Women have modest amounts of DHEA and testosterone in their circulation.[382] It matters to the health of their bones, muscles, and mood. The body uses the molecule DHEA to make testosterone and estrogen. Women worrying about blood sugar clearance may want to know blood levels of both DHEA and testosterone. No need for Rx testosterone gel for women. DHEA supplements are inexpensive and have less risk of over-doing it. There is quite an extensive research literature on use of DHEA supplements in post-menopausal women, and a modest one in men. In one study from 2004, (Journal of American Med Assoc.) DHEA supplements help lower abdominal fat in 56 people, average age 71.[383] In a 2006 paper in the New England Journal of Medicine, DHEA or testosterone didn't help body fat in 83 elderly people. There is no mention of belly fat however. There are some reports of slight improvement in bone mineralization. With blood monitoring of DHEA levels, it is safe.[384] Monitor testosterone levels as well. Excess testosterone is not good, obviously. All in all, DHEA seems to offer only a small possible payoff in helping blood sugar management, and bone mineralization, but I want people to know about it.

Take Care of Bones
Science does not have a full picture on how and why bones play a role in glucose metabolism and insulin messaging. There seems to be some chemical signals that run between fat cells, bone cells and the insulin-producing beta cells of the pancreas.[385] You just want to be sure your bones are doing their best repair work. As you read back on page 103-104, don't rely on drugs for bone health; instead, be authentically nourished. Have plenty of nutrients on hand, in the right amounts, including vit D, vitamin K2, boron and magnesium. Bones not repairing can be from some inflammation going on in the body, and this is likely part of what spills over to insulin issues.

Know Your CRP Level
CRP is often measured as a way to check if someone, with borderline high cholesterol, is at more risk for heart disease. CRP measures inflammation. Higher CRP will suggest that it is "sticky" type, oxidized LDL cholesterol that is circulating in the blood. Higher CRP is an indication that the body is working on cleaning up something, but is having a hard time. Often, just some more B-complex vitamins will support better cell divisions, and lower the CRP. As CRP goes higher, insulin resistance also rises.[386] If higher CRP persists, get some help figuring out what body part is sort of festering, i.e. not successfully repairing.

Initial Diabetes Therapy: Antioxidant-rich diet, plus an antioxidant vitamin
You know that excess inflammation is a big piece of causing insulin resistance. The more antioxidants you have in your diet, the lower the risk and the incidence of insulin resistance. [387] Diet can be potent for reducing inflammation. Some added nutrients, vit C and vit E alone or in combination add some potency to an anti-diabetic scheme. [388 389 390] Animal studies show that the antioxidants are supporting the glutathione (antioxidant) enzyme, and something called H.I.S.S. –Hepatic Insulin Sensitizing Substance. [391] HISS helps insulin talk effectively to muscles. It is best expressed after a meal, versus a snack, and it accounts for 50% of the ability of insulin to deliver its message.[392] While this sounds like a lot of science, I mention it simply as a way to emphasize how dynamic food really is in body processes. Recently, the USDA published the results of a study where the researchers were providing a fruit-fiber-antioxidant bar to people twice a week, for just 2 weeks. They report how glutathione levels started to rise, and inflammation started to go down. It was too short a time to alter insulin function in the study, but when 4 snack bar doses over two weeks are reducing inflammation, it is serious stuff.[393] A fruit-fiber bar is really just you having your fruit-nut caveperson afternoon snack, daily!

Caveman era supplements to help sugar management
I like no-risk nutrient supplements to be therapy for blood sugar problems, before resorting to medications. Sometimes I see a patient who has recently been diagnosed with high blood sugar, but after 3 or 4 weeks of a better diet, neither weight nor blood numbers are coming down the way they should. In this situation, I'll suggest that the person take the amino acid **L-carnitine (1 gram/day)** for a few months.[394] As I mentioned, sometimes cells are clogged with fat, and make themselves insulin-resistant to try to clear out the fat. L-carnitine facilitates fat burning in liver and muscle cells. Unburned fat fragments that are hanging around cells are irritating, and again the irritation causes release of an antagonist to insulin chemical: TNFa if you care to know the name of it. Again, L-carnitine is the gamey-tasting flavor you get in lamb, in moose and elk meat. Exactly, we're not eating gamey-tasting proteins now. You could have mutton (adult sheep) for supper 4 or 5 times a week for a few months, or just take 1 gram L-carnitine a day for 2 months, (2 pills at 500mg each) and help your sugar and weight numbers improve.

The next supplement I'll mention here is **alpha lipoic acid** (ALA). It is also an antioxidant substance.[395] It supports better glutathione levels. You have read enough now to know this will help insulin action. The other fun facet of alpha lipoic acid is that it somehow also helps muscles absorb sugar without needing so much insulin. As insulin delivers "build fat" and make hungry" messages too, less insulin is always nice. Metformin is generally the first drug given to people to manage sugar. A number of people get nausea and other gut side effects from it. I prefer people try ALA. It is a comprehensive antioxidant, so it works to lower risk of nerve and vascular complications caused by high sugar and insulin[396].

Over time, the cells lining arteries get damaged from stray sugar molecules. One form of damage is called "endothelial dysfunction". Arteries receive expand and contract signals for managing blood flow. When an expansion signal shows up, but instead the blood vessels suddenly contract, this is called "endothelial dysfunction". It can cause very high blood pressure. The antioxidant supplement **Co-Enzyme Q10**, at 100mg a day reduces endothelial dysfunction in type 2 DM.[397] This is especially important and useful for people taking "statin" medicine for cholesterol.[398] Remember, I am concerned about an adequate supply of Co Q10 to Natural Killer cells in the Innate Immune system, too.

Diabetes Prescriptions
At some point in diabetes care, you may get started on medicines. You may get started on Metformin (Glucophage), as a pill to help lower sugar. It tries to make insulin receptors be more sensitive. The next drugs used to lower sugar are glipizide (Glucotrol), or glyburide (Micronase & Diabeta). These squeeze more sugar out of pancreatic cells, often causing them to run out of the ability to produce insulin sooner, putting people on a faster course to needing insulin injections. The next step in treatments to manage sugars has been the "glitazone" drugs. It turns out that these convey added cardiac and bladder cancer risks so their use is now curtailed. There was a very deceptive Rosiglitazone paper published in JAIDS in Oct., 2002. The title claimed "Improved Insulin Sensitivity", but the treatment caused dangerous doubling of triglycerides for some subjects.[399] Be very careful if you are taking this drug for diabetes. Other pills and injectibles are coming on the market; each with benefits, but also side effects and cancer risks. The last resort is insulin. While modern insulin therapy is getting easier, with the advent of slow acting, once a day injections with Levemir and Lantus, but being on injections becomes a more complex self-care event. Diabetes is not an easy condition to treat. No pill is as potent as is good diet and exercise.

The Diet For Insulin Resistance
Diets taught to diabetics are still rife with poor advice. Anyone having a diabetic breakfast composed of cereal, milk and banana is tragically misinformed. All three food items digest to become blood sugar, which then requires an insulin response. The triple carb breakfast bowl is absurd. Having the Paleolithic (protein-fruit-nut) breakfast is simply a much lower glucose challenge to the system, plus, it supports better insulin-messaging (H.I.S.S.) action. Keeping insulin expression lower has many benefits. Remember, insulin makes people hungry. So many people with

diabetes complain of constantly craving sugar. The wrong breakfast for a diabetic makes them hungry all day! Careful nutrition to help HISS work better, and then the correct meal composition, will amazingly reverse the sugar cravings.

> Insulin Messages
> 1. Move sugar into cells
> 2. Build fat: make triglycerides
> 3. Retain sodium (raising blood pressure)
> 4. Make hungry / crave sweets

Remember, a diet rich in omega 3 fat, where carbohydrate calories include legumes, and large amounts of vegetable fiber are present is still hugely important.[400] I will once again, make a major plug for eating magnesium-rich foods. See page 40. In a study that watched about 4500 healthy 30 year olds for 20 years, lower magnesium intake was one of the prime conditions in people who developed diabetes![401]

Diabetic Complications

Reversing Diabetic Complications

Neuropathy
Diabetic neuropathy is a common event. Some people with diabetes genes in the family start to develop neuropathy even before they have blood sugar problems. The "thrift gene" that makes people at higher risk for diabetes also causes other metabolism problems. There is a fat processing glitch, where the common LA (linoleic acid) that people get in corn oil and vegetable oil) does not get converted to GLA (**gamma linolenic acid**) well.[402]

There are multiple consequences to the low GLA levels in the body then.

- Cholesterol levels rise, because the enzyme that moves LDL-cholesterol into cells will be low in fuel.
- triglycerides rise
- HDL (good) cholesterol drops.
- Skin can become uncomfortably dry.
- Nerve cells don't repair and start to give a burning feeling, then numbness.

Quite simply, a little known reason for diabetic neuropathy is the essential fat deficiency: low GLA.[403] The American diet can be low in it as people eat mostly processed oils. Most medical providers are unaware of the genetic issues about GLA in Type 2 diabetes.

Taking GLA as supplemental **Evening Primrose Oil (2 grams per day)** may help the neuropathy. Some people use 1 – 2 Tablespoons a day of "cold pressed sunflower seed oil" as a source of GLA too. Borage Oil is also a popular GLA supplement, but I do not recommend it as a GLA supplement, as other substances in borage oil cause "vaso-constriction" ... a shrinking of blood flow in capillaries. This is not en effect you want as a person with diabetes. Primrose oil supplements do not interfere with any medications.

Neuropathy can also occur because of metabolic debris, like free radicals, which can impede circulation. A supplement that is a potent antioxidant that seems to improve circulation in feet is the antioxidant **Alpha Lipoic Acid (ALA)**. [404] It delivers a "grow more capillaries" message in the body too. It works in people with painful neuropathy in their feet. Take 300 mg of Alpha Lipoic Acid, twice a day. **Warning**: blood sugar medicine will likely need adjusting to lower doses when you take ALA. Lipoic acid helps muscles absorb sugar better, so less insulin messaging is needed. Alpha lipoic also helps insulin bind to receptors more effectively.

Benfotiamine for Diabetic Neuropathy
One more nutrient solution known to reverse diabetic neuropathy is benfotiamine. This is a fat-soluble form of Thiamine, which is vitamin B 1, provided in 600 mg a day doses. Trials as 300 mg taken twice a day show better results than one 600 mg dose a day. [405] Take it for 2 months and see how you feel. If it is working, keep going for a few more months.

Being trapped in too many diabetes medicines

I see pharmaceutical company ads on TV, featuring very over-weight women celebrities, speaking for the diabetes drugs that are keeping their blood sugars under control. I see them as people trapped in their fatness, courtesy of the drugs they are pitching. These are affluent people, who are getting the best medical care money can buy. What they are not receiving is smart, functional medicine-type nutritional care.

An example of Alpha Lipoic Acid, Glutamine and other supplements improving blood sugar clearance and reducing insulin needs ....

I once saw an age 50-something woman who was about 100 lbs overweight. For her diabetes, she was taking 85 units of Lantus insulin each evening, and also fast-acting insulin at each meal, adjusting her dose to what her blood sugars were just before eating. (A common Lantus dose may be 20 to 25 units.) She was frustrated that she could not lose weight, no matter how little she ate. She was taking 40 mg of Lipitor a day to knock down cholesterol. Her ankles were generally swollen, as her heart was not pumping strongly enough, so she was also taking furosamide (Lasix), a fluid reduction pill twice a day.

Her frustrations about not losing weight, and her painful swollen ankles had her miserable. She was not all that hungry, and agreed to eat no starches for a few weeks, no bread, rice, pasta, crackers or cereal. Her only carbs were 3-4 small pieces of fruit a day (50 calories each), and the carbs you get in broccoli, spinach, cauliflower and other vegetables (15-40 carb. calories per one or two cup serving). She began the caveperson breakfast: cottage cheese, small apple and 15-20 almonds. Lunch was a huge raw salad, plus salmon or other fish. Snack was a kiwi or dish of berries, plus handful of walnuts or cashews or 2 oz. string cheese. Supper, again, 2 cups of cooked broccoli, spinach, cauliflower or other low calorie vegetables, plus 6 – 8 oz. chicken or lean meat. Evening snack #1 was a low cal yogurt, and #2 was more berries or a Clementine.

Remember, you just read that insulin is a "build fat" message in the body, so of course she was not able to lose weight. Fat cells will only open up and spill their energy to supply fuel in the absence of insulin messaging. I prescribed 300mg Alpha Lipoic Acid pills, one at breakfast, and one at dinner to help cells absorb sugar without needing so much insulin. With the action of the ALA, and the lower carb volume in meals, I warned her to be careful about not taking too much Lantus insulin. Within a day, she no longer needed her fast-acting insulin at meals. Her sugars were lower. Within 10 days, her doctor was lowering her Lantus dose to 55 units!

Time to address the fluid in the ankles too. Remember, Lipitor lowers Co Q10: heart fuel levels. I asked her to take 100 mg Coenzyme Q10, twice a day for a month, and then taper to once a day. This gave her heart more energy, to pump fluid out her legs better. Now, remember, insulin has a "retain sodium" message (by way of its effect on the hormone Aldosterone in the kidney). On the lower carbs food plan, there was less insulin around. On the higher vegetable and correct fruits diet, she was getting more potassium, also pushing sodium out of her body, and fluid levels dropping too. Her ankles were less swollen within a week. Now she was able to lower her Lasix doses too. Within 2 weeks, she was down almost 20 lbs. Yes, this was almost all fluid-weight, but it was a huge psychological boost to someone who was feeling so trapped in her weight.

She was delighted to not have painful, swelling ankles every day. She was psyched to stay on the quite limited food plan, thanks to these results. After a month, her system was working better, so she could "cheat" and dip her vegetables in some humus a few times a week, to add 3 Tablespoons of chickpeas to her salad at lunch.

I had also asked her to use 500 mg L-carnitine twice a day, to be sure her liver could burn fat well. Plus, I had her take L-glutamine, 5 grams a day, to assure optimum insulin messaging at her cells. I am sure you want to know how she did; yes, she lost 100 lbs, in about 9 months.

The point I want to emphasize here is that her medicines were managing symptoms, like high blood sugar, but messing up her metabolism. She was willing to change her diet, and take some more nutritional supplement pills for a few months, to get her system functioning better, and her "disease" status changed radically. She could reduce the medicines that were in the way of her healing. Luckily she had a physician who was willing to work with her, and reduce her meds progressively. The point I want to accent is that the high insulin dose treating her high sugar <u>symptom</u> was preventing weight loss. Food and supplements that treated her insulin resistance <u>problem</u> allowed her to regain her health.

Diabetes in People With HIV

As you know by now, having HIV and/or HCV means there is subtle inflammation happening in various cells throughout the body. Inflammation will generate insulin resistance, which leads to higher blood sugar readings. Simply declaring a higher sugar level in the blood a diabetes condition fails to recognize that some systems are struggling to repair. If you end up just treating the sugar symptom, you fail to fix the underlying problem, and it will go onto to cause troubles in other areas. Shoving more blood sugar into liver and muscle cells will also cause fat and weight accumulation in places you don't want, as well.

When you get the news that your blood sugars are up, start thinking "What system is struggling to repair and sending out distress calls?"

Do a self-scan of your body systems.

How are hormones? Are your testosterone levels OK?
Is Mr. Happy waking up excited a few times a week? If not, this is a sign of low testosterone levels.

Is fitness level ok?
Are your muscles at least a little toned?

How's your waist-hip ratio? Do you get a bloat when you eat?
How about a trial of eating a minimal amount of wheat for 2 weeks?

How are your intestines doing?
Have bowels been too loose for a while?

Are you taking a medicine, like Crestor or another statin,
that causes blood sugar problems? See what probiotics and primrose oil could do for your cholesterol instead (p68). If you could be ok with a lower dose of a statin, that is a better situation.

The Remedies

Maybe you have strayed from you the better food plan that you used to be on. Here is a wake up call, time to get back in gear. Start planning your protein-fruit-nut breakfast.

Time to re-order the good antioxidant vitamins and start taking them.

Time for the fish oils again.

Time to try L-glutamine, 1 teaspoon a day, if you never did before. Time to restart if you ran out a while ago.

Time to get back to doing some fitness activity, too; a yoga class, some routine walking, maybe a splurge on a swim club membership?

A Few Words About Caring For The Liver

Having your liver in its best state of repair matters to so many systems in the body. Watching LFT's ... liver function tests ... is how medical people monitor the liver. When the ALT and/or AST numbers rise, you want to know why, and see if the culprit can be eliminated. One common reason for higher ALT is Hepatitis C infection. I have written a whole book about nutritional care for people with Hep C, People wanting more detailed knowledge can get that book. Meanwhile, I will just provide a short account of liver support in general here.

Brief Science Lesson about Liver Metabolism

Remember glutathione enzyme (GSH) is the major antioxidant peptide (protein) scavenging free radicals in the liver. Its cousin glutathione peroxidase (GSX) is also very busy in some viral infections.[406] Both vitamin C and vitamin E are "glutathione-sparing" which means they try to grab free radicals first, leaving less work for GSH.[407] In a study that was following over 130 HIV-infected injection drug using people in New York, people who maintained higher GSH levels live longer.[408] I have previously mentioned, in either HCV or HIV infection, many studies document lower level GSH activity: in lungs,[409] in liver,[410] and in circulating immune cells.[411] Interestingly, too, in the mix of HCV and HIV infection, plus protease inhibitor treatment, it is still the medicine that is most responsible for liver irritation.[412]

Food And Supplements That Support Liver Repair

Dietary support for repair of the liver starts with a high quality protein diet. Then comes antioxidant support of the liver. Then there is CD8 cell support in the form of adequate vitamins and minerals that support antiviral activity in the liver.

As LFT's improve, a person might be able to drop the volume of antioxidant support for Glutathione. Alpha Lipoic Acid, NAC, and glutamine overlap in their Glutathione support. Maintain one of those items, even once ALT and AST are closer to normal.

In other pages, I have emphasized glutathione support, especially after age 50. There are implications for immune support and good T cell function,[413] stronger Th1 response--CD8 cell activity,[414] and prevention of T cell depletion.[415] Glutathione support with NAC has improved outcomes in Hep B,[416] and Hep C treatments.[417] Better levels have implications for preventing emphysema in poz smokers.[418] The best liver support is broad in scope. It all starts with lifestyle moves though, as the Herzenbergs point out in their paper showing that supporting glutathione improves survival: abstaining from drugs and alcohol, and improving diet can all help raise glutathione levels and improve LFT's.[419]

Using L-glutamine in a fragile liver.

A clinical note: I am always trying to provide needed nutrients to any struggling cell system. These days, people are more often dieing of liver failure than they are of HIV disease it self. I always try to repair liver cells whenever possible. I have used glutamine supplementation, even in late liver disease, and have remarkable success. It takes several weeks to see results, because what is happening is glutathione level improvement happens first, then, this enables more liver cell repair.

In case you need an in depth look into liver metabolism of ammonia, read Glutamine and Hepatic Metabolism in <u>Organ Metabolism and Nutrition: Ideas for Future Critical Care.</u> Edited by Kinney and Tucker, Raven Press, Ltd. New York 1994.)

"The affinity for ammonium ions for urea synthesis in the liver periportal circulation is lower than that of glutamine synthetase in the perivenous circulation."

People with compromised livers, who are on a protein restriction, might try 5 grams of glutamine for 3 – 4 weeks to see if they can actually improve liver function. Their ammonia levels do not worsen, so after 4 weeks, add 5 more grams of glutamine and and LFT's start to come down more. Have some L-carnitine with this too. Do not do this at home though. Have professional monitoring. Carnitine reverses hepatic encephalopathy too, better than lactulose, without the diarrhea issues of lactulose.

It is just so important to keep the liver healthy.

When The Liver is Struggling, Muscle Repair Will Be Neglected

(The next page here is designed to be a quick easy handout for helping people take care of their liver.) Copy and distribute it as needed.

Food & Supplements For Liver Repair   charlienutrition.com

Every day, eat a diet that includes:

1. Protein foods at breakfast, lunch and dinner
2. Fruit servings 3-4 times per day
3. Vegetables, at least 2 cups a day
4. Carbohydrates that digest slowly
5. Fats that do not clog your body

Don't get stressed out if this seems like you will have to make too many changes in how you eat. Just start somewhere and make progress over the months. You are still supposed to enjoy lots of good food. Here are some easy changes you might start with.

- Lean ham replaces fatty sausage in a breakfast sandwich
- Ground turkey replaces beef hamburger in spaghetti sauce or lasagna.
- An apple and a handful of walnuts replace candy as an afternoon snack.
- Pork chops instead of steak for dinner, much less iron and fat.

Take some vitamins and other supplements to keep your liver in great shape.

Step 1. Shop www.vitaminshoppe.com or www.newyorkbuyersclub.org for supplements

An enhanced **iron-free** multivitamin that includes adequate amounts of magnesium, zinc, vit D & selenium for immune cell support. Extra antioxidants, especially vitamin E and vitamin C, to prevent inflammation.	Two Per Day Tablets multivitamin by Life Extension Foundation, or Perfect Family Iron-free, (3+/day), by Supernutrition. Or Active 50+ Once Daily from Trader Joes.

Step 2.

Glutathione support, as extra liver repair material, immune cell support and added antioxidant power, especially if ALT is >80.	NAC (n-acetylcysteine) 1 gram per day L-glutamine powder, 5 grams (1 teasp): each taken once or twice per day.

Step 3

Mitochondrial support, to restore or boost energy	L-carnitine: 1-2 grams per day Co-enzyme Q10: 100 mg per day.

Do Step 1 all the time, and then do Steps 2 & 3, either continuously, or as needed.

A day of good eating:
Breakfast: whey protein-fruit smoothie, or cottage cheese and fruit, & handful of walnuts.
Snack: oatmeal with milk, or rye toast with some nut butter.
Lunch: sardines or salmon on a salad with black beans or rye crackers, olive oil in the dressing.
Snack: trail mix; or some fruit and a handful of nuts or seeds.
Dinner: fish, chicken, turkey or pork, baked potato or peas, lots of vegetables.
Snack: more fruit; plus a low fat, low sugar yogurt

People going on Interferon/Ribavirin/Protease therapy should do Steps 1-3 for 2-4 weeks before starting treatment; and continue. They will have much fewer side effects. For my Hep C nutrition book, shop at: www.eatupbooks.net .

Lipodystrophy Is Still Happening

While the exact origin of lipodystrophy has not been nailed down, there are many snap shot pictures of it that give clues for managing or reducing it. People without HAART get lipopystrophy, which suggest some elements of infection cause it. Elevations in the cytokines TNFa [420] and IFNa [421] exist in lipodystrophy, pointing to inflammation as a cause. Nucleoside drugs are an issue as you just read, so mitochondrial toxicity contributes. Then, factor in protease inhibitor therapy, through the effects of PI's on fat cell genetics and insulin-GLUT4 signaling.[422] In reality, it is a blend of diet, plus all these parameters that is the issue.

For a simplistic argument however, think about food versus medicines for a minute. People might take 40 milligrams a day of Stavudine/D4T, while they consume 80,000 milligrams of triglyceride a day, and 350,000mg of glucose/starch. Now ask yourself, "Which might have more impact on fat and cholesterol and body shape?" Then consider, a one-hour brisk walk may burn 17000 mg of fat too. While there may be just a little leeway in choice of medicines; there can be a great deal of movement in dietary manipulation. Food does play a dynamic role in modulating metabolism and body shape. For example, going on a high carbohydrate diet for weight loss tends to cause a loss of fat mostly from the area below the waist, whereas a lower carb diet will promote fat loss from the upper body.[423] This is a very simplistic argument, but people in lipodystrophy research studies, like Dr. Grinspoon's at Massachusetts General Hospital, report to me that while in the study, the medicines or exercise programs worked a little bit, but once they cleaned up their diet, the medicines really helped their lipodystrophy problem. Remember, good food is powerful.

DON'T LET THIS DOWNWARD SPIRAL HAPPEN TO YOU!

Avoid the downward spiral of throwing prescription medications at lipodystrophy symptoms before nutritional bases are covered. Too often Lipitor is used to treat elevated cholesterol and TG's (blood lipids). This fails to treat the free fatty acid (FFA) problem in muscle and liver mitochondria that provoked the blood lipid problem. Further accumulation of FFA's provokes more TNFa cytokine release and promotes insulin resistance. Blood sugars rise, and then a "glitazone" diabetes medicine like Actos or Avandia is prescribed. It often does not adequately solve blood glucose problems, so insulin is prescribed. On insulin, a person ends up making more triglycerides so their numbers rise to 700 or 1000!!! Very scary. All the fat swirling in the blood causes even more protease paunch! This is a heart attack in the development, despite a ton of modern medicines. In this scenario, a person is doing fine with HIV, but is now at great risk for pancreatitis and heart attack. The downward spiral all started because of a failure to treat the fat dysmetabolism at its fundamental source: mitochondrial distress.

Muscles and Mitochondrial Toxicity

Muscles are also very much affected by the anti-HIV medicines called nucleoside analogues. Muscle disturbances from nucleoside analogue medicines (AZT, D4T, 3TC, ddI, ddC etc) were described as far back as 1990 in the New England Journal of Medicine.[424] An expert detail of the science of the nucleoside irritation in nerves and muscles comes in *Nature Medicine* back in 1995.[425] The trend is to use more *nucleotide* medicine now, not *nucleosides,* and in much lower doses than in the early 1990's. However, there is no proof that the body suddenly recovers to normal function. For example, in a "switch study" when people were moved from AZT etc., to tenofovir therapy, triglyceride numbers dropped just 0.5 mmol/L, which is about 44 milligrams.[426] At the same time, medicines are less toxic now, but being on them for 10 or 15 years means even a little hassle can accumulate. The stray electrons of daily living add to mitochondrial irritation, too. Even tenofovir/Viread bothers glutathione levels in mitochondria. [427]

The Mitochondria story

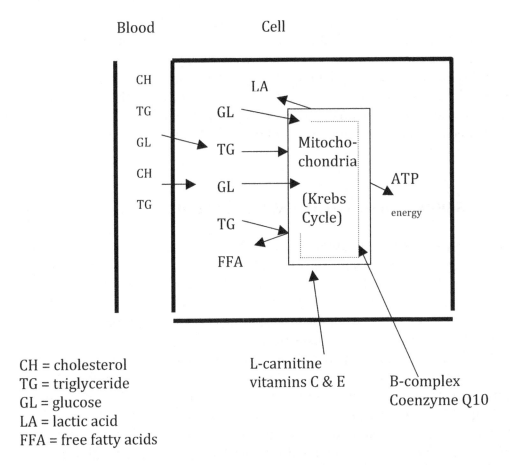

CH = cholesterol
TG = triglyceride
GL = glucose
LA = lactic acid
FFA = free fatty acids

Glucose (sugar) and Triglyceride (fat) move from the blood into cells, but then must move into the mitochondria (oven) to be converted into ATP (energy). Stray electrons, nucleoside meds like AZT, D4T and Trizavir corrode the oven walls. The

Hepatitis C virus itself, and the nucleoside drug Ribavirin are both toxic to liver cell mitochondria too. First effect, energy/ATP production is slower, so people can feel a little sluggish. Over a longer period of time, fat stops moving through the mitochondrial walls as easily as it should. Bits of fat (free fatty acids) accumulate in the interior of the cell. [428] Fat accumulation here is a big piece of the start of lipodystrophy.

The stray extra fat droplets, --free fatty acids--- cause insulin resistance.[429] The concept is that the cells are burning less fat and more sugar. In this scenario, more lactic acid is being made. (Same as you pedaling a bike up hill and feeling your thighs burn.) If too much lactic acid were to happen, the whole body would become acidic, and very sick. The body compensates, then, by "resisting" the insulin message next time that it comes along to tell a cell to absorb more sugar. If sugar is not moving, the pancreas puts out even more insulin with the result being hyperinsulinemia.[430] Hyper insulinemia is associalted with higher TG's in the blood too. So one of the main issues in lipodystrophy is keeping mitochondria is good shape.

Keeping Mitochondria In Good Condition

The combination of stray electrons from HIV infection, plus the stress of nucleosides produce a measurable effect on mitochondria. The combination of Vitamin C at 1000mg/day and vitamin E at 600iu/day can cut that stress in half, and restore mitochondria to full function. [431] Remember, when cell damage accumulates, cytokine messages increase. Excess free fatty acids inside cells causes TNFa levels to rise. Mitochondria that are irritated by oxidative stress also invoke cytokines.

Cytokines, themselves, cause a disruption in fat burning. The message of TNFa and IFNg is to toss more free fatty acids into the fuel mix, and inhibit insulin action. So cytokines will also disrupt usual fat clearance. Eating the wrong fats in the diet, not getting enough omega 3 fish oils in food, excesses of sugar, plus not getting enough protein, will promote excess cytokine activity. Exercise, that reduces the excess fat in muscles, lowers TNFa levels.[432] Exercise improves body fat status too.[433] Your goal is to keep fat metabolism going in the right ways.

Exercise plus smart vitamins and adequate dietary protein are the key ingredients for keeping mitochondria in best fuel-processing condition.

Rx LIPODYSTROPHY .... FOCUS ON FAT METABOLISM IN MITOCHONDRIA

At the first sign of elevated cholesterol, or body shape changes, go looking for elevations in triglycerides. The TG (VLDL) molecule travels in the blood with a cholesterol coating, and this is often what raises serum cholesterol. Before worrying about egg yolks and shrimp and dietary cholesterol, think about food: fats and carbohydrates. Revert to cave man cuisine.

After intestines and liver, muscles are the place where the side effects of HIV infection and its drug treatment most hit people. Myalgias (aches) and fatigue should be assessed and treated. Nutrition is the treatment of choice.

I want people to have a sense that all options may still be open when they are hoping to recover from some old side effects from their anti-HIV treatment. There are no hopeless cases. It could be years since you stopped AZT, it is still worth a few months of supplements to see what further rehab of muscles or nerves could be accomplished. For some people, it is happening that they need to revisit taking Combivir(AZT) because of bone or kidney issues with Tenofovir/Viread, and they're concerned about AZT side effects. No worries, just support mitochondria in muscles, nerves and the liver.

I recall a middle-aged man patient I saw years ago, He was on therapy with Kaletra and Fortovase (no nucleoside at this point). Because his blood fat numbers were high, his MD had him also taking 10 mg of Lipitor. When he came to see me, his Cholesterol was 278 and his triglycerides were 1700! His diet was good, except 1 dark chocolate bar in the afternoon, 'cause he felt an energy slum at that time of day.

When you see high triglycerides think mitochondrial rehab and cleaner diet.

Well, his protease inhibitors were slowing sugar clearance and previous Combivir had slowed fat-burning in muscles. His mitochondria needed help, even though he was no longer on an antagonistic therapy. It was a multivitamin, fish oils and L-carnitine to the rescue. In 7 weeks time, his triglycerides dropped to 166, and cholesterol to 172. He said he was inspired to eat some more fruit and vegetables when he heard me lecture about caveman diet. He also admitted to feeling motivated to use a treadmill for a few walks a week. About 6 months later I saw him again. He said he was less diligent about restricting chocolate and using the treadmill, but his cholesterol and triglyceride numbers were still fine. Again, it was mitochondrial rehab that allowed him to have good blood fat numbers, despite being less restrictive with his diet.

Reduce Your Risk Of Getting Diabetes Along With Your Lipodystrophy

You read earlier about subtle inflammation as a something that provokes diabetes. High triglycerides are sometimes a suggestion that your HAART drugs are increasing your blood sugar, and have you pointed in the diabetes direction. You can reduce diabetes risk. Glucose is managed by insulin. Insulin works with glucose tolerance factor (GTF). GTF is composed of Glutathione, Niacin, & Chromium. [434] Over time, you can expect your chromium levels to be low due to malabsorption. Take 200 mcg chromium/day for 1 month. Niacin is part of the B-complex you are taking. Taking 1 gram of NAC/day plus 5 grams of glutamine helps maintain good glutathione levels. Alpha lipoic acid also helps keep glutathione levels higher at 300mg, taken twice a day.

Pick some glutathione support supplement and take it for a month or two.

Insulin receptor status on muscles is a function of "in-shape" level of muscles, and repair status. Do some resistance training exercise: this means lifting weights.

Testosterone levels also impact sugar processing and storage in liver. Have your free testosterone levels checked every 6 months if you are worried about your metabolism, especially if your TG's are high.

Remember, if worried about blood sugar levels, think about improving fat metabolism and reducing inflammation first. A clinical picture to appreciate: Dr. Steve Grinspoon described the presence of excess free fatty acids in lipodystrophy.[435] He blocked their release with acipomox, and glucose metabolism improved.[436] His colleague Colleen Hadigan described how higher intakes of polyunsaturated fats is part of lipodystrophy.[437] She thought that perhaps excesses of trans fat was the issue, but in fact, corn oil, vegetable oil and the polyunsaturated fats are inflammatory and irritating compounds. These modern, industrial fats can stimulate fat cell production, in both good and bad ways.[438] Dr. Gelato tried insulin sensitizers in some HIV+ people at risk for diabetes. While the title of her article claims insulin function got better, [*Improved insulin sensitivity and body fat distribution in HIV-infected patients treated with rosiglitazone: a pilot study*], the consequences were quite undesirable. In the data of the article, triglycerides rose in 5 of 8 people in her study, even doubling in two people, 174 to 410, and 669 to 1548![439] Hidden in the fine print of this study is one person who dropped out due to elevated LFT's! Rosiglitazone treatment is known to cause liver failure. So 1 of 9 did not complete the "study" here. This was a deceptive article title. While insulin action seemed to improve, the clinical result was bad news. Remember, sometimes the liver is insulin-resistant for a reason. It is trying to not burn sugar, so don't go using drugs to ram more sugar in. You can get dangerous levels of triglycerides as a result.

The point of the story here is that insulin receptors are not the primary problem in HIV-related glucose problems. Asking peripheral fat cells to suck up stray fat droplets (FFA's) is not the way to go. [440] [441] Some peripheral lipase sluggishness and higher gut-area fat are operating behind the scenes.[442] Remember, the trouble is provoked by hypermetabolism and by lack of nutrients. Focus on better fat clearance in mitochondria.

Lipodystrophy is about clogged fat metabolism in liver and muscle cells.

I cannot emphasize enough the combined role of fish oils[443] and antioxidant vitamins and a period of L-carnitine therapy[444] as the important first steps in treating lipodystrophy, and reversing blood sugar and high triglyceride problems in HIV care.

Your Lipodystrophy Treatment Roadmap (as of 2014)

1. Be on a caveman-era diet, which supports and does not stress all aspects of body and T cell repair; and does not create energy processing hassles. Follow a diet with extra protein, correct fats, and quality starch choices and portions.
2. Take some antioxidant and B-complex vitamins to keep mitochondria in muscles and nerves buffed up.
3. Engage in some muscle-toning exercise; if more time is available, also do some cardio exercise.
4. At first sign of fat metabolism troubles, take 3 grams a day of fish oils.
5. Add some glutathione/liver support supplement if needed, like NAC/glutamine or alpha lipoic acid.
6. Take 1 gram of L-carnitine each day for 2 – 3 months.
7. Be sure testosterone is up to functional levels.

Your nutritional strategy is to eat wisely, and take a few vitamins to be in great shape. Sometimes you might need to take some other supplements for a month or two to get your metabolism back in order.

One brilliant concept that simply gets no airplay in discussion of lipodystrophy is that there appears to be a **constant autonomic nervous system activation** that is redirecting metabolism.[445] Why no attention to this? It is most likely because there is no drug treatment that could be promoted to manage it. The autonomic nervous system is what restores balance and equilibrium in body systems. Being nourished helps the balance. Eastern modalities, accupuncture, Tai Chi and Tong Ren energy healing help the autonimic nervous system though. Again, see page 133 to learn about accessible Tong Ren energy medicine treatment.

Infection, Medicines and Sideeffects

Here is a review of a few symptoms people have that affect quality of life. Often nutritional therapy can provide some relief.

Trouble-shooting symptoms

Tiredness and fatigue remedy ...

Be sure you are eating 3/4 your ideal weight in grams of protein. If not already taking some, start taking a daily B-complex 25 vitamin. Take a 100 mg Coenzyme Q10 pill twice a day, every day, for three to four weeks. This helps most people. If these help some, but not quite enough, then add 5 grams a day of L-glutamine too. Last supplement to try would be 1 gram per day of L-carnitine.

Abdominal bloat and gas within 15 minutes of eating a meal...

Try having no wheat for a week. This means: no pasta, bread, noodles, toast, crackers, muffins, etc. for 7 days. If this is helpful, see your doctor for gluten-sensitivity blood tests. Even if gluten intolerance is not the diagnosis, you could still have "wheat sensitivity". Many people are finding they just don't do well with wheat. It doesn't matter if it is white wheat, sprouted wheat or whole wheat; the current hybridized form of wheat grown around the globe is bothering many people. Read the book *The Wheat Belly Diet*, by cardiologist William Davis, MD for more details.

Nausea and body/gut distress

Nausea in the HAART era is likely a side effect of medicines bothering the liver. Taking 1 gram NAC and 5 grams L-glutamine for a few weeks generally remedies the nausea. This was a lifesaver for people in 1996, trying to cope with Norvir therapy and vomting three times a day for weeks while their liver acclimated to the drug.

Consider checking lactic acid levels. Yes, you might have good T cells and low viral load, and lactic acid problems! Symptoms are fatigue, nausea, and aches.

Nerves Are Vulnerable, And Their Nutrient Supply Is Hurting.

Nerve problems in HIV disease mostly come as a side effect from antiviral drug treatment, particularly the nucleoside analogue drugs. Nerve cells are thought to never repair, but that concept needs revisiting in the context of mitochondrial toxicity. The nutrients most responsible for nerve health are some most likely to be deficient in HIV disease: L-Carnitine, Co-enzyme Q10, vitamin B-12, and magnesium.

Over time, it seems that the infection affects nerves of the brain. It is still too soon to tell whether this is malnutrition, toxicity of meds, or innate damage due to immune activation or infiltration by immune cells. What is known though, is that supplements well past the RDA for B-vitamins do improve mood.[446] [447]

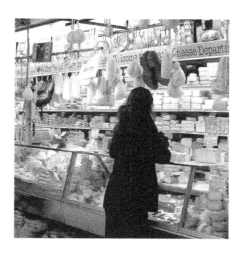

Reducing Neuropathy

Medicines treating neuropathy only block pain, and don't stop the damage cells may be experiencing. The set of supplements listed here is worth trying to see if they could reduce irritation and nerve pain. Try them for 2 months to see if you get help. While nerve cells that are damaged for too long may not repair, I have had a number of patients with chronic pain, not relieved by heavy doses of Neurontin, get great benefit from this nutritional intervention. **This treatment is focused on lessening mitochondrial distress, and providing key repair nutrients generally low in HIV+ people.**

Magnesium deficiency in the nervous system allows toxic chemicals to accumulate in nerve cells and damage them.[448] Take **400 mg/day magnesium** to help prevent more damage. **Magnesium sulfate** is the best form to take.[449]

Everyone with HIV disease should be taking B-complex vitamins, but if you have neglected yours lately, get back on them. A **B-complex 25 or B-complex 50 pill once a day** is a good amount to take. **Methylcobalamin** is the best form of vitamin B-12 to have in the B-complex pill.[450] The Jarrow Company makes **B Right** a B-complex with methycobalamin as the B-12 source; otherwise by a B-12 lozenge.

The nervous system can run low on vitamin B-12 before the vitamin shows up deficient in the blood system. A daily **1 mg B-12 pill** loads your system. Again, methylcobalamin lozenges are a good way to get the B-12. Yes, take this in addition to the B-12 in the B-complex pill. There is no toxic dose of B-12.

When you have painful neuropathy, try extra vitamin B-6, pyridoxine.[451] Buy a bottle of **100 milligrams B-6 pills**. Take **2 per day,** spread out over the day. (Yes, take these in addition to your other B-complex and B-12 pills.) Take the B-6 for 8 weeks at the most. Once your nerves are feeling better, stop the extra B-6 and just continue your B-complex pill and B-12 lozenge. Taking B-6 at 400 mg doses can damage nerves. Just take the two 100mg pills for 8 weeks.

The amino acid **L-carnitine** helps activate B-12 for better action in repairing nerve cells. It also reduces mitochondrial distress. Taking **1 or 2 grams of L-carnitine per day** can reduce neuropathy pain. Use this for 8 weeks as well. In some areas, Carnitor (the prescription form) is paid for by insurance. Remember, taking 2 grams L-carnitine for lowering triglycerides above the 1000 level is a good idea.

Coenzyme Q10 also helps improve mitochondrial energy production. Taking **100mg Coenzyme Q10 per day** completes the panel of neuropathy reversing supplements. If money is limited, taking it even 10 days or two weeks helps. Then just 2-3 times a week would help if that is all that is affordable.

The antioxidant **alpha lipoic acid** is commonly used to treat the pain of diabetic neuropathy in Europe. Doses run from 400 mg to 1800 mg per day. Lipoic acid seems to improve circulation into nooks and crannies of cells of the body.[452] How much it contributes to actual nerve repair I am not sure, so I don't usually recommend it in this neuropathy treatment. Other people do, at 400 mg per day. However, I still do like it for liver support and for treatment of diabetic neuropathy.

If your previous medical treatment had you using a "d" drug, like D4T, or ddI, and you have lingering neuropathy, you might try vitamins and carnitine for 2 months. Take a B-12 pill and a B-complex vitamin each day. Take 1 gm Carnitine daily as well. Also, if you consume alcohol, drink only in moderation for a while, 1 or 2 drinks, just a few times a week.

Many people also have good results using acupuncture to relieve pain of neuropathy. Don't worry; the acupuncture needles don't hurt. Acupuncture helps reduce a lot of HIV disease symptoms. Again, I will mention that I have had tremendous success with these supplements and Tong Ren energy healing combined.

Energy Healing With Tong Ren Therapy

Eastern medicine includes a concept that the flow of essential energy is a key component of health and wellbeing. The energy is called Chi, or Qi, pronounced "chee". Chi is supposed to be running all through the body, from head to toe. We are all made up of atoms, organized into molecules, clumped into constructs like organs and bones. Food is also a collection of atoms and molecules. Remember, atoms have a nucleus containing protons, with electrons spinning around them. The body parts also have orbiting electrons. Well, lets just imagine that sometimes the energy frequency of various electrons can sometimes be just slightly out of synchronicity. In this situation, maybe the food you eat won't quite be absorbed into some cells as well as it could. Maybe the electrons of your hormone insulin will be slightly out of orbit, so it won't stimulate muscle cells as functionally as it needs to.

Eastern medicine practitioners direct the flow of Chi (coming down from high in the sky) through the body, to get all electrons and body parts back into harmony or synchronicity. The benefit may be that chi flow is simply getting all the nutrients of broccoli or any other food, to fully absorb into and nourish cells. All this happens when both food and body energy systems are in their correct orbits.

The synchronicity concept extends to having body systems in tune as well. You want the electrons / energy pattern of your T cells, to be in synch with your lymph flow for maximum delivery of antiviral activity.

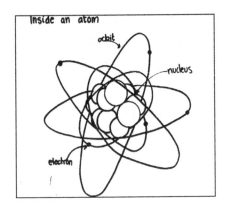
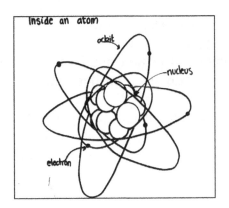

broccoli atoms   muscle cell atoms

There are a number of ways to get Chi flowing. People can do organized, patterned, movement sequences like tai chi and chi gung. Acupuncture works too. Tuina massage and cupping also get Chi flowing. These modalities are all wonderful, but can cost a lot for individual treatments, or require a lot of learning to do the tai chi movements correctly.

I want people to know about **Tong Ren energy healing**. It is totally non-invasive: no touching, no needles, no pills. A Tong Ren practitioner uses mental focus to direct energy to the recipient, to get Chi flowing. How the practitioner focuses is tapping on parts of an acupuncture teaching doll, or on a diagram/drawing that illustrates acupuncture points. The recipient simply sits quietly and receives energy. Some telepathy, or communication utilizing the Jungian collective unconscious occurs, and the recipients feel some heat or tingling, as their Chi flows a little better. Once Chi is moving, the body's own repair materials move better. Many remarkable improvements happen. Arthritis pain is diminished, nerves feel calmer, and headaches lessen. Tong Ren is a wonderful accompaniment to nutritional care. I put people on a diabetic diet, and ask them to let me do 5 minutes of Tong Ren energy work with them. When they are back in my office in 3 weeks, they are losing weight and their blood sugars are normal and they are feeling better. Part of the success of Tong Ren therapy is a change in brain wave energy flow. My colleague William Daley, MD descibes this brain activity in the next few paragraphs.[453] (at www.tomtam.com)

Brainwave Entrainment For Synchronicity.
The animal kingdom demonstrates a capacity we share. The perfectly synchronized movements of birds flying in a flock, or fish swimming in a school are not coordinated by the usual senses of sight, sound, smell, feel or taste -- but rather by "brainwave entrainment" with an instinctive commonality. They move in perfect harmony because each is connected with the brainwave energy and patterns of the group. A natural propensity toward synchronization is even seen in non-biologic systems, such as two pendulum clocks side-by-side on a wall gradually moving into harmony. The human brain has a Frequency Following Response, tending to change

its dominant electroencephalogram patterns toward the frequency of external stimuli. Several studies have demonstrated a strong tendency for brainwaves of meditating people to synchronize with each other, with no sensory contact.
Dr. Carl Jung, Pierre Teilhard de Chardin, Ervin Laszlo, Gary Zukav and others have described the evolving development of a subconscious human connectedness, like a global spirit or brain. As an anthropologist, Teilhard traced the natural evolution of life on earth from the development of cells, then plants, through animal and finally human form. This visible biologic evolution then progressed to internal intellectual development, and now finally to globally evolving organization on the level of spirit-energy. We are all part of this upward spiral of organization, regardless of our awareness. In Tong Ren Therapy we tap into this vast reserve of healthy bioelectrical patterns and health-sustaining energy. We then use the natural tendency toward synchronicity to bring diseased organs back into harmony with the healthy bioelectric patterns of Tong Ren practitioners, and even more importantly into entrainment with the more powerful global brain.

I have had nice results using a blend of some vitamins or other supplements with Tong Ren. I have improved T cell counts by 200 points. I have reversed long-standing neuropathies. For something that is non-invasive and inexpensive, I think it is worth pursuing. The Spaulding Rehab Hospital, a division of Mass General Hospital, has Sunday afternoon Tong Ren healing classes in Boston. Spinal cord injury and stroke patients are finding the sessions helpful. Watch a broadcast sometime, at www.tongrenstation.com. Sit at your computer screen, hands in your lap. Give it a few tries. See www.TongRenNutrition.org for some short therapeutic sessions too.

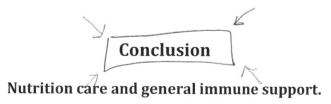

Conclusion

Nutrition care and general immune support.

HIV care in an ageing population means acting in a world with less than perfect knowledge. Good care still demands paying attention to processes that are at risk. HIV care clinicians are confronted with managing many familiar events in an ageing population. Cholesterol and maybe triglyceride numbers are rising; blood pressure numbers are too. Bones are thinning. There is insulin resistance or frank diabetes to control also.

The previous discussion here has hopefully shed some light on nutritional processes that are happening in both ageing and chronic infection. It is important to remember, medicines are not appropriate or effective treatment for nutritional deficiencies. When diabetes is happening because of excessive inflammation, the standard insulin receptor interventions for treatment simply won't be as efficacious, and could produce undesired results. What will happen is poly-pharmacy for problems with poor results, frustrating both patients and providers. Becoming comfortable and skillful with a modest list of nutritional supplements for common conditions can have a dynamic, beneficial, impact on HIV care for people as they progress in years.

Failure to address the nutritional pathologies places patients at unnecessary risk. Excess redox burden raises risk for thromboses. Excess TNFa expression is connected to cART failure. Diet must still be stressed as fundamental to HIV care. Tossing a statin drug at a cholesterol problem may leave a person at risk for immune deficiency, due to excess sat fat in the diet. Stronger statin doses increase the chance of diabetes, in a population that already has more risk.

Therapeutic lifestyle needs to be accented as fundamental to HIV care for people as they age. Besides all its benefits on body and mind, exercise slows the fundamental mechanism of ageing: the shortening of telomeres. Exercise impacts weight, which impacts redox load. Good nutrition impacts antiviral capacity of the body, and is the only available treatment of immune senescence. In addition to food and dietary elements, nutrient supplements are needed to address the inflammatory state. Helping patients make lifestyle changes takes continuous motivational support. Intervening with nutrition generally meets with good compliance, since the pills have good effects, and no undesirable side effects. My goal is that people using all the information presented here end up feeling stronger and more energetic, and have clear clinical improvements.

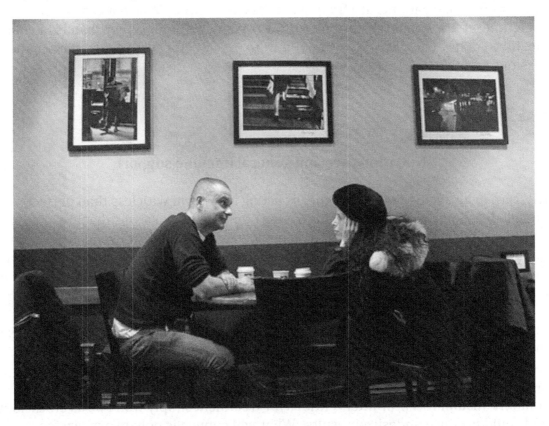

Special thanks to Karen Larsen for wonderful photos.[454]

Appendix #1
Supporting Immune, Muscle, Liver and other Cells

1) Your system is growing new T cells by the millions every week. You need extra vitamins and protein for this.
2) The debris from used-up T cells is now scattered around. These stray electrons are called "free radicals" and can damage other cells if not captured and tamed. Anti-oxidant systems in your body clean up the stray electrons, otherwise you get inflammation, liver damage, and fat redistribution problems.
3) Anti-HIV medicines irritate many cells and these need some repair too. Meds are a bit less toxic, so I am lowering the minimum levels that people may need.

Here are the nutrients studied in HIV care, and at what doses.

Antioxidant vitamins are:	vitamin C 500 mg	1 or 2 per day
	Vitamin E 200 iu.	1 or 2 per day
	(Best if Vit E is "mixed tocopherols.)	
	Beta carotene 20,000 iu a day, <u>in food</u>	
Antioxidant minerals are:	selenium 200 mcg	1 or 2 per day
	magnesium 200 mg	1 or 2 per day
Liver repair vitamins are:	B-complex 25 or 50	1 pill a day
Liver repair amino acids are:	N-acetylcysteine 1 to 2 grams a day	
	L-glutamine (GLN) 5 to 10 grams a day	
	Take GLN, 10 grams, 2 – 3 X a day for problematic diarrhea	
Essential fat:	Evening Primrose Oil 2 grams a day	
	EPA/DHA Omega 3 fish oils 2 – 5 gms/day	
Energy that Liver exports:	Co-enzyme Q10 100mg 1 or 2 per day	
Mitochondrial toxicity repair:	L-Carnitine 1 to 2 gms a day for 1-2 mo.	
Body Cell Mass Repair:	Agrinine/Glutamine/HMB -- Juven – 2 /day	

Don't get overwhelmed by this list. It is all the possible nutrient therapies you could utilize. It is unlikely that you'd need them all at once. See next section.

Appendix #2
Practical Supplement Intervention

If your diet is quite nourishing, these 3 supplements will cover you. Take: the **Supernutrition Simply One 50+** multivitamin, 1 teaspoon a day lof **L-glutamine**, and a 100 mg **Co-enzyme Q10** pill a day. You will be in great shape.

Here in detail are some other choices ....

1. **Enhanced Multivitamin**: 100% RDA for usual vitamins, 100 mg Magnesium, 100 mcg Selenium, plus 10 X RDA B-complex, vit C & E.

Examples:
Simply One 50+ Mens Vitamin by Supernutrition, Whole Foods $25/mo
Simply One 50+ Womens Vitamin by Supernutrition, Whole Fds $25/mo
Active Senior Multivitamins by Rainbow Light   Vit Shoppe $9
Two Per Day Tablets* by Life Extension   Vit Shoppe $ 8.50
Active 50+ Once Daily Multivitamin & Mineral   Tr. Joe's $ 5
 (you will pee yellow from these vitamins, from the Stress Tab part)

2. **Essential Fatty Acids** & phospholipids   Vit Shoppe or Trader Joe's
Maintain arterial health, & peripheral lipase and nitric oxide functions.

Omega 3 EPA/DHA fatty acids: > 800 mg/day as 2-3 gms **Fish Oils**
   (4 oz. salmon or 3.5 sardines, etc. is approx. 1700 mg EPA/DHA)
   Trader Joe's EPA/DHA 500 or Nordic Naturals products

Omega 6 GLA **Evening Primrose Oil**: 1000 – 1300 mg pill, take 2 per day
   Fixes dry skin caused by diabetes genes & raises good HDL cholesterol.
   1000mg Trader Joe's and 1300 mg The Vitamin Shoppe

3. **Glutathione support**   The Vitamin Shoppe
   Helps lung & liver irritation, supports insulin, helps grow muscle

1- 2 gms NAC ... N-acetylcysteine **NAC**
5 grams **L-glutamine**   (1 round teaspoon powder)
(w/ glutamine: **JarroDophilus eps**, probiotic, for intestine repair; 2/day)

4, **Mitochondrial Rehabilitation.** for 2-3 months ....
   Helps reduce Triglycerides and reverse neuropathy & fatigue

L-carnitine 1 gram per day   The Vitamin Shoppe
Co-enzyme Q10 100 mg, 1/day   Trader Joes

Appendix #3 — **Guide To Groceries**

REPAIR FOODS	ANTIOXIDANT & IMMUNE SYSTEM FOODS		ENERGY FOODS	
PROTEINS	**VEGES**	**FRUITS**	**STARCHES**	**FATS OILS**
Salmon	Carrots	Oranges	**Black beans**	Walnuts
Sardines	**Broccoli**	**Bananas**	**Red kidney b.**	**Almonds**
Herring	**Spinach**	*Grapefruit*	**White kidney b.**	Pecans
Trout	Winter squash		**Lentils**	Brazil nuts
Cod	**Kale**	Apricots	**Chick peas**	Cashews
Haddock	**Swiss chard**	Cantaloupe	**Black-eyed peas**	Pistachio nuts
Flounder	**Collard greens**	Clementines	**Navy beans**	Pine nuts
Shrimp		Mangos	**Lima beans**	Macadamia nuts
Scallops	Asparagus	Nectarines		Ground flax
Lobster	Beets	Papaya	Quinoa	seeds
Tuna	Brussels sprouts	Peaches	**Sweet potatoes**	
	Cabbage	Pomegranate	Yams	
DesignrWhey	Cauliflower	**Blueberries**	Peas	Sunflower seeds
Protein	**Dark lettuce**	**Strawberries**	Corn	Pumpkin seeds
No fat/Low fat	Eggplant	**Raspberries**	Plantain	Sesame seeds
cott. cheese	Green beans	Red grapes	Potatoes	
Egg whites	Green peppers	Honeydew	Buckwheat	Olives
Vege. Burger	Red peppers	Watermelon		Avocado
Turkey breast	Mushrooms	Kiwis	Oatmeal	
Turkey ham	Mustard greens	**Apples**	Cheerios	Soy nuts
Turk. sausage	Okra	**Applesauce**	Oat Bran	Peanuts /oil
Chicken breast	Pea Pods	**Pears**	Corn tortillas	
Chicken legs	**Tomato sauce**	Pineapple	Rye bread 100%	**Olive oil (ideal)**
Chicken thighs	Turnip	Plums	Brown rice	
Pork tenderloin	Celery			Smart Balance/
Pork chop	Onion	Dates	*(careful)*	Olivio/
Lite/low fat	Parsnip	Figs	*Whole wheat*	tub margarine
cheeses	Summer squash	Raisins	*bread* (reflux)	Butter
Omega 3 eggs	Zucchini squash	Cran-raisins	Spaghet/noodles	Canola oil
Lamb Chops	Cucumbers	Lychee	White bread	
Grass-fed:			Bagels	*(avoid)*
Hamburger	**Calcium foods**	(4 oz. juices)	White rice	Corn oil
Round steak	Low fat milk	apricot nectar	Muffins	Vegetable oil
Sirloin steak	Yogurt	pineapple jce	Waffles	Fried fast foods
Filet	Almond milk	grapefruit jce	Pancakes	Stick margarine
	Algaecal .com	orange juice	Cookies	
	supplement	pom. juice	Cakes	

Using The Guide To Groceries: foods in BOLD print are extra nourishing

The Protein Column
Eat protein at breakfast as well as lunch and supper. Fish at the top, with omega 3's are super good for you. Yes, they are brain food, and prevent heart attacks. Seafood is fine, but have it cooked, not raw. Shrimp and lobster don't contain a lot of cholesterol. Research has figured out that there are useful many plant sterols that actually lower cholesterol. Chicken and turkey are ok too; they have little fat. Lean pork is fine too; it is the other white meat these days. Moving to beef, just keep to the lean items, like a sirloin steak; **grass fed** would be extra good. Dairy fat is controversial for people worried about cholesterol; low fat dairy products are ok though. Eggs are totally fine, buy omega 3 eggs if you can; the chickens were fed better. Milk and yogurt come low fat; they are just a 1/2 size portion of protein. They have about 8 or 10 grams of protein per serving, and you are usually looking for 20 - 30 grams at a meal. Add a scoop of **Designer whey** protein powder to make the milk in your cereal be a full protein serving. It's also helps bones and liver repair.

The Vegetable Column
All vegetables are great. The ones at the top of the list just happen to be extra nutritious. They have more carotenes, or more potassium, or both, plus other minerals. Eat vegetables at both lunch and dinner.

The Fruit Column
All fruits are good. The ones at the top of the list just happen to be extra nutritious. They have more vitamin C, or more potassium, or both. Eat fruit 3 or 4 times a day. The **Fruits** are the ones that help brain cells work better.

The Starch Column
Eating more foods from the top of the list is a great idea. Notice that beans are really a starch. 80% of their calories come from carbohydrate, and just 20% from protein. Then eat yams, peas, corn, and plantain. Next, eat whole grains. Rye is <u>much</u> better than wheat. The foods at the top of the column cause the slowest blood sugar rise. The foods at the bottom have the least vitamins and minerals, plus added bad news grease and sugar.

The Oils Column
A handful of nuts and one of seeds each day is good for your health. As much as possible, have the oil that goes into your body be more from the foods like nuts and seeds, plus from fish. Cook with olive oil. Notice that corn oil, safflower oil, vegetable oil are low on the list; they are somewhat inflammatory. Smart Balance tub margarine tastes and acts like butter, but does not hurt your cholesterol. Enjoy butter, but in modest amounts, for special foods.

As you assemble meals, think about having some Repair food (protein), some Immune Support (veges or fruit) and then some Energy foods (a starch and fat mix). Even with all these great foods, take an antioxidant vitamin for best health.

REFERENCES

[1] Muller FL, Lustgarten MS, Jang Y, Richardson A, Van Remmen H. Trends in oxidative aging theories. Free Radic Biol Med. 2007 Aug 15;43(4):477-503.

[2] Schumacher B, van der Pluijm I, Moorhouse MJ et al. Delayed and accelerated aging share common longevity assurance mechanisms. PLoS Genet. 2008;4(8):e1000161.

[3] Pérez VI, Bokov A, Van Remmen H, Mele J, Ran Q, Ikeno Y, Richardson A. Pérez VI, Bokov A et al. Is the oxidative stress theory of aging dead? Biochim Biophys Acta. 2009;1790(10):1005-14.

[4] Weber TA, Reichert AS. Impaired quality control of mitochondria: aging from a new perspective. Exp Gerontol. 2010 Aug;45(7-8):503-11.

[5] Rebrin I, Sohal RS. Pro-oxidant shift in glutathione redox state during aging. Adv Drug Deliv Rev. 2008;60(13-14):1545-52.

[6] Gorbunova V, Seluanov A. Making ends meet in old age: DSB repair and aging. Mech Ageing Dev. 2005;126(6-7):621-8.

[7] Kim J, Sapienza CM. Implications of expiratory muscle strength training for rehabilitation of the elderly: Tutorial. J Rehabil Res Dev. 2005;42(2):211-24.

[8] Abdelhafiz AH, Brown SH, Bello A, El Nahas M. Chronic kidney disease in older people: physiology, pathology or both? Nephron Clin Pract. 2010;116(1):c19-24.

[9] Biagi E, Nylund L, Candela M, et al. Through ageing, and beyond: gut microbiota and inflammatory status in seniors and centenarians. PLoS One. 2010;5(5):e10667.

[10] Tiihonen K, Ouwehand AC, Rautonen N. Human intestinal microbiota and healthy ageing. Ageing Res Rev. 2010;9(2):107-16.

[11] Sawabe M. Vascular aging: from molecular mechanism to clinical significance. Geriatr Gerontol Int. 2010. Suppl 1:S213-20.

[12] Ponnappan S, Ponnappan U. Aging and immune function: Molecular mechanisms to interventions. Antioxid Redox Signal. 2011;14(8):1551-85.

[13] Sansoni P, Vescovini R, Fagnoni F, Biasini C, Zanni F, Zanlari L, Telera A, Lucchini G. et al. The immune system in extreme longevity. Exp Gerontol. 2008;43(2):61-5.

[14] Effros RB, Dagarag M, Spaulding C, Man J. The role of CD8+ T-cell replicative senescence in human aging. Immunol Rev. 2005;205:147-57.

[15] Alberti S, Cevenini E, Ostan R, Capri M, Salvioli S, Bucci L, Ginaldi L, De Martinis M. et al. Age-dependent modifications of Type 1 and Type 2 cytokines within virgin and memory CD4+ T cells in humans. Mech Ageing Dev. 2006;127(6):560-6.

[16] Effros RB. Telomerase induction in T cells: a cure for aging and disease? Exp Gerontol. 2007;42(5):416-20.

[17] Xu Q, Parks CG, DeRoo LA, Cawthon RM, Sandler DP, Chen H. Multivitamin use and telomere length in women. Am J Clin Nutr. 2009;89(6):1857-63.

[18] Harley CB, Liu W, et al. A Natural Product Telomerase Activator As Part of a Health Maintenance Program. Rejuvenation Res. 2011;14(1):45-56

[19] Kirk JB, Goetz MB. Human immunodeficiency virus in an aging population, a complication of success. J Am Geriatr Soc. 2009;57(11):2129-38.

[20] Taiwo B, Hicks C, Eron J. Unmet therapeutic needs in the new era of combination antiretroviral therapy for HIV-1. J Antimicrob Chemother. 2010;65(6):1100-7.

[21] Desai S, Landay A. Early immune senescence in HIV disease. Curr HIV/AIDS Rep. 2010;7(1):4-10.

[22] Ances BM, Ortega M, Vaida F, Heaps J, Paul R. Independent effects of HIV, aging, and HAART on brain volumetric measures. JAIDS. 2012;59(5):469-77.

[23] Becker JT, Maruca V, Kingsley LA, Sanders JM, Alger JR, Barker PB, Goodkin K, Martin E et al. Multicenter AIDS Cohort Study Factors affecting brain structure in men with HIV disease in the post-HAART era. Neuroradiology. 2012;54(2):113-21.

[24] Maggi P, Serio G, Epifani G, Fiorentino G, Saracino A, Fico C, Perilli F, Lillo A, Ferraro S, Gargiulo M et al. Premature lesions of the carotid vessels in HIV-1-infected patients treated with protease inhibitors. AIDS. 2000;14(16):F123-8.

[25] De Socio GV, Martinelli C, Ricci E, Orofino G et al; HERMES study group. Relations between cardiovascular risk estimates and subclinical atherosclerosis in naive HIV patients: results from the HERMES study. Int J STD AIDS. 2010;21(4):267-72.

[26] Dressman J, Kincer J, Matveev SV, Guo L, Greenberg RN, Guerin T, Meade D, Li XA, Zhu W et al. HIV protease inhibitors promote atherosclerotic lesion formation independent of dyslipidemia by increasing CD36-dependent cholesteryl ester accumulation in macrophages. J Clin Invest. 2003;111(3):389-97.

[27] Alter G, Altfeld M. NK cells in HIV-1 infection: evidence for their role in the control of HIV-1 infection. J Intern Med. 2009;265(1):29-42.

[28] Solana R, Tarazona R, Gayoso I, Lesur O, Dupuis G, Fulop T. Innate immunosenescence: Effect of aging on cells and receptors of the innate immune system in humans. Semin Immunol. 2012 Oct;24(5):331-41.

[29] Hatano H, Delwart EL, Norris PJ, Lee TH, Neilands TB, Kelley CF, Hunt PW, Hoh R, Linnen JM, Martin JN et al. Evidence of persistent low-level viremia in long-term, HAART-suppressed, HIV-infected individuals. AIDS. 2010;24(16):2535-9.

[30] Famularo G, Moretti S, Marcellini S, Alesse E, De Simone C. Cellular dysmetabolism: the dark side of HIV-1 infection. J Clin Lab Immunol. 1996;48(3):123-32.

[31] Herzenberg LA, De Rosa SC, Dubs JG, Roederer M, Anderson MT, Ela SW, Deresinski SC, Herzenberg LA. Glutathione deficiency is associated with impaired survival in HIV disease. Proc Natl Acad Sci U S A. 1997;94(5):1967-72.

[32] Morbitzer M, Herget T. Expression of gastrointestinal glutathione peroxidase is inversely correlated to the presence of hepatitis C virus subgenomic RNA in human liver cells. J Biol Chem. 2005;280(10):8831-41.

[33] Ogunro PS, Ogungbamigbe TO, Elemie PO, Egbewale BE et al. Plasma selenium concentration and glutathione peroxidase activity in HIV-1/AIDS infected patients: a correlation with the disease progression. Niger Postgrad Med J. 2006;13(1):1-5.

[34] Ofori H, Jagodziński PP. Increased in vitro replication of CC chemokine receptor 5-restricted human immunodeficiency virus type 1 primary isolates in Th2 lymphocytes may correlate with AIDS progression. Scand J Infect Dis. 2004;36(1):46-51.

[35] Becker Y. The changes in the T helper 1 (Th1) and T helper 2 (Th2) cytokine balance during HIV-1 infection are indicative of an allergic response to viral proteins that may be reversed by Th2 cytokine inhibitors and immune response modifiers--a review and hypothesis. Virus Genes. 2004;28(1):5-18.

[36] Fraternale A, Paoletti MF, Dominici S, Buondelmonte C, Caputo A, Castaldello A, Tripiciano A, Cafaro A, Palamara AT et al. Modulation of Th1/Th2 immune responses to HIV-1 Tat by new pro-GSH molecules. Vaccine. 2011;29(40):6823-9.

[37] Skurnick JH, Bogden JD et al. Micronutrient profiles in HIV-1-infected hetero-sexual adults. J Acquir Immune Defic Syndr Hum Retrovirol. 1996;12(1):75-83.

[38] Aukrust P, Müller F, Lien E, Nordoy I, Liabakk NB, Kvale D et al. Tumor necrosis factor (TNF) system levels in human immunodeficiency virus-infected patients during highly active antiretroviral therapy: persistent TNF activation is associated with virologic and immunologic treatment failure. J Infect Dis. 1999;179(1):74-82.

[39] Lacey JM, Wilmore DW. Is glutamine a conditionally essential amino acid? Nutr Rev. 1990;48(8):297-309.

[40] Dröge W, Schulze-Osthoff K, Mihm S, Galter D, Schenk H, Eck HP, Roth S, Gmünder H. Functions of glutathione and glutathione disulfide in immunology and immunopathology. FASEB J. 1994;8(14):1131-8.

[41] Multhoff G, Meier T, Botzler C, Wiesnet M, Allenbacher A, Wilmanns W, Issels RD. Differential effects of ifosfamide on the capacity of cytotoxic T lymphocytes and natural killer cells to lyse their target cells correlate with intracellular glutathione levels. Blood. 1995;85(8):2124-31.

[42] Rahman I, MacNee W. Oxidative stress and regulation of glutathione in lung inflammation. Eur Respir J. 2000 Sep;16(3):534-54.

[43] Marí M, Morales A, Colell A, García-Ruiz C, Fernández-Checa JC. Mitochondrial glutathione, a key survival antioxidant. Antioxid Redox Signal. 2009;11(11):2685-700.

[44] Lei XG, Cheng WH, McClung JP. Metabolic regulation and function of glutathione peroxidase-1. Annu Rev Nutr. 2007;27:41-61.

[45] Wanchu A, Rana SV, Pallikkuth S, Sachdeva RK. Short communication: oxidative stress in HIV-infected individuals: a cross-sectional study. AIDS Res Hum Retroviruses. 2009 Dec;25(12):1307-11.

[46] Levent G, Ali A, Ahmet A, Polat EC, Aytaç C, Ayşe E, Ahmet S. Oxidative stress and antioxidant defense in patients with chronic hepatitis C patients before and after pegylated interferon alfa-2b plus ribavirin therapy. J Transl Med. 2006 Jun 20;4:25.

[47] Baum MK, Sales S, Jayaweera DT, Lai S, Bradwin G, Rafie C, Page JB, Campa A. Coinfection with hepatitis C virus, oxidative stress and antioxidant status in HIV-positive drug users in Miami. HIV Med. 2011;12(2):78-86.

[48] Vendemiale G, Grattagliano I, Portincasa P et al. Oxidative stress in symptom-free HCV carriers: relation with ALT flare-up. European J Clin Investigation 2001 31(1):54-63.

[49] Ko WS, Guo CH, Yeh MS, Lin LY, Hsu GS, Chen PC, Luo MC, Lin CY. Blood micronutrient, oxidative stress, and viral load in patients with chronic hepatitis C. World J Gastroenterol. 2005;11(30):4697-702.

[50] Lee MH, Yang HI, Lu SN, Jen CL, Yeh SH, Liu CJ, Chen PJ, You SL, Wang LY, Chen WJ, Chen CJ. Hepatitis C virus seromarkers and subsequent risk of hepatocellular carcinoma: long-term predictors from a community-based cohort study. J Clin Oncol. 2010;28(30):4587-93.

[51] Tanaka H, Fujita N, Sugimoto R, Urawa N, Horiike S, Kobayashi Y, Iwasa M, Ma N, Kawanishi S, Watanabe S, Kaito M, Takei Y. Hepatic oxidative DNA damage is associated with increased risk for hepatocellular carcinoma in chronic hepatitis C. Br J Cancer. 2008;98(3):580-6.

[52] Wen CP, Lin J, Yang YC, Tsai MK, Tsao CK, Etzel C, Huang M, Hsu CY, Ye Y, Mishra L, Hawk E, Wu X. Hepatocellular carcinoma risk prediction model for the general population: the predictive power of transaminases. J Natl Cancer Inst. 2012;104(20):1599-611. doi: 10.1093/jnci/djs372.

[53] Guo CH, Chen PC, Lin KP, Shih MY, Ko WS. Trace metal imbalance associated with oxidative stress and inflammatory status in anti-hepatitis C virus antibody positive subjects. Environ Toxicol Pharmacol. 2012;33(2):288-96.

[54] Kato J, Kobune M, Nakamura T, Kuroiwa G, Takada K, Takimoto R, Sato Y, Fujikawa K, Takahashi M, Takayama T, Ikeda T, Niitsu Y. Normalization of elevated hepatic 8-hydroxy-2'-deoxyguanosine levels in chronic hepatitis C patients by phlebotomy and low iron diet. Cancer Res. 2001 Dec 15;61(24):8697-702.

[55] Kobayashi H, Matsuda M, Fukuhara A, Komuro R, Shimomura I. Dysregulated glutathione metabolism links to impaired insulin action in adipocytes. Am J Physiol Endocrinol Metab. 2009;296(6):E1326-34.

[56] Neuman RB, Bloom HL, Shukrullah I, Darrow LA, Kleinbaum D, Jones DP, Dudley SC Jr. Oxidative stress markers are associated with persistent atrial fibrillation. Clin Chem. 2007;53(9):1652-7.

[57] Evereklioglu C, Er H, Doganay S, Cekmen M, Turkoz Y, Otlu B, Ozerol E. Nitric oxide and lipid peroxidation are increased and associated with decreased antioxidant enzyme activities in patients with age-related macular degeneration. Doc Ophthalmol. 2003;106(2):129-36.

[58] Mondal D, Pradhan L, Ali M, Agrawal KC. HAART drugs induce oxidative stress in human endothelial cells and increase endothelial recruitment of mononuclear cells: exacerbation by inflammatory cytokines and amelioration by antioxidants. Cardiovasc Toxicol. 2004;4(3):287-302.

[59] Sekhar RV, Patel SG, Guthikonda AP, Reid M, Balasubramanyam A, Taffet GE, Jahoor F. Deficient synthesis of glutathione underlies oxidative stress in aging and can be corrected by dietary cysteine and glycine supplementation. Am J Clin Nutr. 2011;94(3):847-53.

[60] http://changingminds.org/explanations/needs/maslow.htm

[61] O'Keefe JH Jr, Cordain L. Cardiovascular disease resulting from a diet and lifestyle at odds with our Paleolithic genome: how to become a 21st-century hunter-gatherer. Mayo Clin Proc. 2004;79(1):101.

[62] Gaffney-Stomberg E, Insogna KL, Rodriguez NR et al. Increasing dietary protein requirements in elderly people for optimal muscle and bone health. J Am Geriatr Soc. 2009;57(6):1073-9.

[63] Willett W. Fruits, Vegetables, and Cancer Prevention: Turmoil in the Produce Section. J Natl Cancer Inst 102(8): 510-11.

[64] Sponheimer M, Lee-Thorp JA. Isotopic evidence for the diet of an early hominid, Australopithecus africanus. Science. 1999;283(5400):368-70.

[65] Wolever TM, Mehling C. Long-term effect of varying the source or amount of dietary carbohydrate on postprandial plasma glucose, insulin, triacylglycerol, and free fatty acid concentrations in subjects with impaired glucose tolerance. Am J Clin Nutr. 2003;77(3):612-21.

[66] Iannuzzi-Sucich M, Prestwood KM, Kenny AM. Prevalence of sarcopenia and predictors of skeletal muscle mass in healthy, older men and women. J Gerontol A Biol Sci Med Sci. 2002;57(12):M772-7.

[67] Frank R, Berndt ER, Donohue J, Epstein A, Rosenthal M. Trends in Direct-to-Consumer Advertising of Prescription Drugs. Kaiser Family Foundation Document. 2002.

[68] Simopoulos AP, Visioli F. More on Mediterranean Diets. World Review of Nutrition and Dietetics, Vol 97: P 68. Karger 2007

[69] Simopoulos AP. Evolutionary aspects of diet: the omega-6/omega-3 ratio and the brain Mol Neurobiol. 2011;44(2):203-15

[70] David Heber, MD PhD. *What Color Is Your Diet?* Regan Books/Harper Collins, 2001.

[71] Kimm SY, Glynn NW, Aston CE, Damcott CM et al. Racial differences in the relation between uncoupling protein genes and resting energy expenditure. Am J Clin Nutr. 2002;75(4):714-9.

[72] Uribarri J, Cai W, Peppa M, Goodman S, Ferrucci L, Striker G, Vlassara H. Circulating glycotoxins and dietary advanced glycation endproducts: two links to inflammatory response, oxidative stress, and aging. J Gerontol A Biol Sci Med Sci. 2007;62(4):427-33.

[73] Saraswat M, Reddy PY, Muthenna P, Reddy GB. Prevention of non-enzymic glycation of proteins by dietary agents: prospects for alleviating diabetic complications. Br J Nutr. 2009;101(11):1714-21.

[74] Hurst S, Rees SG, Randerson PF, Caterson B, Harwood JL. Contrasting effects of n-3 and n-6 fatty acids on cyclooxygenase-2 in model systems for arthritis. Lipids. 2009;44(10):889-96.

[75] Min Y, Lowy C, Islam S, Khan FS et al. Relationship between red cell membrane fatty acids and adipokines in individuals with varying insulin sensitivity. Eur J Clin Nutr. 2011;65(6):690-5.

[76] Smith WL. Cyclooxygenases, peroxide tone and the allure of fish oil. Curr Opin Cell Biol. 2005;17(2):174-82.

[77] Merino DM, Ma DW, Mutch DM. Genetic variation in lipid desaturases and its impact on the development of human disease. Lipids Health Dis. 2010. 18;9:63.

[78] Schubert R, Kitz R, Beermann C, Rose MA, Lieb A, Sommerer PC et al. Effect of n-3 polyunsaturated fatty acids in asthma after low-dose allergen challenge. Int Arch Allergy Immunol. 2009;148(4):321.

[79] Tapiero H, Ba GN, Couvreur P, Tew KD. Polyunsaturated fatty acids (PUFA) and eicosanoids in human health and pathologies. Biomed Pharmacother. 2002 Jul;56(5):215-22.

[80] Stoll AL, Locke CA, Marangell LB, Severus WE. Omega-3 fatty acids and bipolar disorder: a review. Prostaglandins Leukot Essent Fatty Acids. 1999;60(5-6):329-37.

[81] Frisardi V, Panza F, Seripa D, Imbimbo BP, Vendemiale G, Pilotto A, Solfrizzi V. Nutraceutical properties of Mediterranean diet and cognitive decline: possible underlying mechanisms. J Alzheimers Dis. 2010;22(3):715-40.

[82] Conquer JA, Holub BJ. Supplementation with an algae source of docosahexaenoic acid increases (n-3) fatty acid status and alters selected risk factors for heart disease in vegetarian subjects. J Nutr. 1996;126(12):3032-9.

[83] http://www.amazon.com/s/?ie=UTF8&keywords=dha+gummy&tag=googhydr-20&index=aps&hvadid=12499647107&ref=pd_sl_4kwisxtzfu_b

[84] Yurko-Mauro K. Cognitive and cardiovascular benefits of docosahexaenoic acid in aging and cognitive decline. Curr Alzheimer Res. 2010;7(3):190-6.

[85] SanGiovanni JP, Chew EY, Agrón E et al. Age-Related Eye Disease Study Research Group. The relationship of dietary omega-3 long-chain polyunsaturated fatty acid intake with incident age-related macular degeneration: AREDS report no. 23. Arch Ophthalmol. 2008;126(9):1274-9.

[86] Hibbeln JR, Nieminen LR, Blasbalg TL, Riggs JA, Lands WE. Healthy intakes of n-3 and n-6 fatty acids: estimations considering worldwide diversity. Am J Clin Nutr. 2006;83(6 Suppl):1483S-1493S.

[87] Gesch CB, Hammond SM, Hampson SE, Eves A, Crowder MJ. Influence of supplementary vitamins, minerals and essential fatty acids on the antisocial behaviour of young adult prisoners. Randomised, placebo-controlled trial. Br J Psychiatry. 2002;181:22-8.

[88] Freeman MP, Hibbeln JR, Wisner KL, Davis JM, Mischoulon D, Peet M, Keck PE Jr, Marangell LB, Richardson AJ, Lake J, Stoll AL. Omega-3 fatty acids: evidence basis for treatment and future research in psychiatry. J Clin Psychiatry. 2006;67(12):1954-67.

[89] William Evans, PhD & Irving Rosenberg, MD, *Biomarkers*. Fireside, 1992.

[90] Vergel N, Mooney M. *Built To Survive.* 2003

[91] Campbell WW, Trappe TA, Wolfe RR, Evans WJ. The recommended dietary allowance for protein may not be adequate for older people to maintain skeletal muscle. J Gerontol A Biol Sci Med Sci. 2001;56(6):M373-80.

[92] Marco V. Narici†* and Nicola Maffulli. Sarcopenia: characteristics, mechanisms and functional significance. British Medical Bulletin 2010; 95: 139–159.

[93] Janssen I, Heymsfield SBet al. Low relative skeletal muscle mass (sarcopenia) in older persons is associated with functional impairment and physical disability. J Am Geriatr Soc. 2002; 50(5):889-96.

[94] Kotler DP, Tierney AR, Wang J, Pierson RN Jr. Magnitude of body-cell-mass depletion and the timing of death from wasting in AIDS. Am J Clin Nutr. 1989;50(3):444-7.

[95] O'Keefe JH Jr, Cordain L. Cardiovascular disease resulting from a diet and lifestyle at odds with our Paleolithic genome: how to become a 21st-century hunter-gatherer. Mayo Clin Proc. 2004;79(1):101-8.

[96] Evans WJ. Protein nutrition, exercise and aging. J Am Coll Nutr. 2004; 23(6 Suppl):601S-609S.

[97] Paddon-Jones D. Rasmussen BB. Dietary protein recommendations and the prevention of sarcopenia: Protein, amino acid metabolism and therapy. Curr Opin Clin Nutr Metab Care. 2009; 12(1): 86–90.

[98] Iglay HB, Apolzan JW, Gerrard DE, Eash JK, Anderson JC et al. Moderately increased protein intake predominately from egg sources does not influence whole body, regional, or muscle composition responses to resistance training in older people. J Nutr Health Aging. 2009;13(2):108-14.
[99] Albert CM, Hennekens CH, O'Donnell CJ, Ajani UA, Carey VJ, Willett WC, Ruskin JN, Manson JE. Fish consumption and risk of sudden cardiac death. JAMA. 1998 ;279(1):23-8.
[100] Donald R. Davis, PhD, FACN, Melvin D. Epp, PhD et al. Changes in USDA Food Composition Data for 43 Garden Crops, 1950 to 1999 Journal of the American College of Nutrition, 2004. 23:(6): 669–682.
[101] United Kingdom, Medical Research Council, Ministry of Agriculture: Royal Society of Chemistry; http://www.mineralresourcesint.co.uk/pdf/mineral_deplet.pdf .
[102] Hibbeln JR. From homicide to happiness--a commentary on omega-3 fatty acids in human society. Cleave Award Lecture. Nutr Health. 2007;19(1-2):9-19.
[103] Selhub J, Jacques PF, Bostom AG, D'Agostino RB, Wilson PW, Belanger AJ, O'Leary DH, Wolf PA, Schaefer EJ, Rosenberg IH. Association between plasma homocysteine concentrations and extracranial carotid-artery stenosis. N Engl J Med. 1995;332(5):286-91.
[104] Johansson M, Relton C, Ueland PM, et al. Serum B vitamin levels and risk of lung cancer. JAMA. 2010 Jun;303(23):2377-85.
[105] Fawzi WW, Msamanga GI, Spiegelman D, Urassa EJ, McGrath N, Mwakagile D, Antelman G, Mbise R et al. Randomised trial of effects of vitamin supplements on pregnancy outcomes and T cell counts in HIV-1-infected women in Tanzania. Lancet. 1998;351(9114):1477-82.
[106] Baum MK, Mantero-Atienza E, Shor-Posner G, Fletcher MA, Morgan R, Eisdorfer C, Sauberlich HE, Cornwell PE, Beach RS. Association of vitamin B6 status with parameters of immune function in early HIV-1 infection. J Acquir Immune Defic Syndr.;4(11):1122-32.
[107] Altura BM, Altura BT. Magnesium and cardiovascular biology: an important link between cardiovascular risk factors and atherogenesis. Cell Mol Biol Res. 1995;41(5):347-59.
[108] Durlach J, Bac P, Durlach V, Rayssiguier Y, Bara M, Guiet-Bara A. Magnesium status and ageing: an update. Magnes Res. 1998;11(1):25-42.
[109] Skurnick JH, Bogden JD, Baker H, Kemp FW, Sheffet A et al. Micronutrient profiles in HIV-1-infected heterosexual adults. J Acquir Immune Defic Syndr Hum Retrovirol. 1996;12(1):75-83.
[110] Beck KW, Schramel P, Hedl A, Jaeger H, Kaboth W. Serum trace element levels in HIV-infected subjects. Biol Trace Elem Res. 1990;25(2):89-96.
[111] Rylander R, Mégevand Y, Lasserre B, Amstutz W, Granbom S. Moderate alcohol consumption and urinary excretion of magnesium and calcium. Scand J Clin Lab Invest. 2001;61(5):401-5.
[112] Holick MF. Calcium and Vitamin D. Diagnostics and Therapeutics. Clin Lab Med. 2000 Sep;20(3):569-90.
[113] Lips P, Bouillon R, et al. Reducing fracture risk with calcium and vitamin D. Clin Endocrinol (Oxf) 2010; 73(3):277-85.
[114] Dawson-Hughes B. Serum 25-hydroxyvitamin D and muscle atrophy in the elderly. Proc Nutr Soc. 2012; 71(1):46-49.
[115] Kampman MT, Steffensen LH. The role of vitamin D in multiple sclerosis. J Photochem Photobiol B. 2010;101(2):137-41.
[116] Porojnicu AC, Robsahm TE, Dahlback A et al. Seasonal and geographical variations in lung cancer prognosis in Norway. Does Vitamin D from the sun play a role? Lung Cancer. 2007;55(3):263-70.
[117] Holick MF. Vitamin D and sunlight: strategies for cancer prevention and other health benefits. Clin J Am Soc Nephrol. 2008;3(5):1548-54.
[118] Khokhar JS, Brett AS, Desai A. Vitamin D deficiency masquerading as metastatic cancer: a case series. Am J Med Sci. 2009;337(4):245-7.
[119] Cannell JJ, Vieth R, Umhau JC, Holick MF, Grant WB, Madronich S, Garland CF, Giovannucci E. Epidemic influenza and vitamin D. Epidemiol Infect. 2006;134(6):1129-40.
[120] Berry DJ, Hesketh K, Power C, Hyppönen E. Vitamin D status has a linear association with seasonal infections and lung function in British adults. Br J Nutr. 2011;106(9):1433-40.
[121] Cannell JJ, Zasloff M, Garland CF, Scragg R, Giovannucci E. On the epidemiology of influenza. Virol J. 2008;5:29.
[122] Aloia JF, Li-Ng. Correspondence, Re: Epidemic Influenza and Vitamin D. Epidemiol Infect. 2007; 135(7): 1095–1098.
[123] Simonsen L, Taylor RJ, Viboud C, Miller MA, Jackson LA. Mortality benefits of influenza vaccination in elderly people: an ongoing controversy. Lancet Infect Dis. 2007;7(10):658-66.
[124] Yao X, Hamilton RG, Weng NP, Xue QL, Bream JH, Li H, Tian J, Yeh SH, Resnick B, Xu X, Walston J, Fried LP, Leng SX. Frailty is associated with impairment of vaccine-induced antibody response and increase in post-vaccination influenza infection in community-dwelling older adults. Vaccine. 2011;29(31):5015-21.
[125] Wouters-Wesseling W, Rozendaal M, Snijder M, Graus Y, Rimmelzwaan G, De Groot L, Bindels J. Effect of a complete nutritional supplement on antibody response to influenza vaccine in elderly people. J Gerontol A Biol Sci Med Sci. 2002;57(9):M563-6.
[126] Meydani SN, Meydani M, Blumberg JB, Leka LS, Siber G, Loszewski R, Thompson C, Pedrosa MC, Diamond RD, Stollar BD. Vitamin E supplementation and in vivo immune response in healthy elderly subjects. A randomized controlled trial. JAMA. 1997;277(17):1380-6.
[127] Fraternale A, Paoletti MF, Casabianca A, Oiry J, Clayette P et al. Antiviral and immunomodulatory properties of new pro-glutathione (GSH) molecules. Curr Med Chem. 2006;13(15):1749-55.
[128] Stey C, Steurer J, Bachmann S, Medici TC, Tramèr MR. The effect of oral N-acetylcysteine in chronic bronchitis: a quantitative systematic review. Eur Respir J. 2000;16(2):253-62.
[129] Decramer M, Rutten-van Mölken M, Dekhuijzen PN, Troosters T, van Herwaarden C, Pellegrino R, van Schayck CP, Olivieri D, Del Donno M et al. Effects of N-acetylcysteine on outcomes in chronic obstructive pulmonary disease (Bronchitis Randomized on NAC Cost-Utility Study, BRONCUS): a randomised placebo-controlled trial. Lancet. 2005;365(9470):1552-60.
[130] Weatherall M, Clay J, James K, Perrin K et al. Dose-response relationship of inhaled corticosteroids and cataracts: a systematic review and meta-analysis. Respirology. 2009;14(7):983-90.

[131] Dröge W, Holm E. Role of cysteine and glutathione in HIV infection and other diseases associated with muscle wasting and immunological dysfunction. FASEB J. 1997;11(13):1077-89.

[132] Julius M, Lang C, Gleiberman L, Harbijrg E, et al. Glutathione and morbidity in a community-based sample of elderly. ClinEpidemiol 1994. 47: (9)1021-1026.

[133] Bengmark S. Econutrition and health maintenance: A new concept to prevent inflammation, ulceration and sepsis. Clin Nutr 1996;15:1-10.

[134] Andrew Weil, MD Spontaneous Healing, Balantine Books, 1995, pp156-9.

[135] Castro-Giner F, Künzli N, Jacquemin B, Forsberg B, de Cid R, Sunyer J, Jarvis D, Briggs D, Vienneau D, Norback D, González JR, Guerra S, Janson C, Antó JM et al. Traffic-related air pollution, oxidative stress genes, and asthma (ECHRS). Environ Health Perspect. 2009;117(12):1919-24.

[136] Wood LG et al. Reduced circulating antioxidant defenses are associated with airway hyper-responsiveness, poor control and severe disease pattern in asthma. Br J Nutr. 2010;103(5):735-41.

[137] Produce For Better Health Foundation; The State of America's Plate 2005: study on America's Consumption of Fruit and Vegetable. AC Neilsen, 2004 survey. PBH Foundation, 7465 Lancaster Pike Suite J, 2nd Floor, Hockessin, DE 19707

[138] Simopoulos AP. Evolutionary aspects of omega-3 fatty acids in the food supply. Prostaglandins Leukot Essent Fatty Acids. 1999; 60(5-6): 421-9.

[139] Stampfer MJ, Hennekens CH, Manson JE, Colditz GA, Rosner B et al. Vitamin E consumption and the risk of coronary disease in women. N Engl J Med. 1993;328(20):1444-9.

[140] Pfister R, Sharp SJ, Luben R, Wareham NJ, Khaw KT. Plasma vitamin C predicts incident heart failure in men and women in European Prospective Investigation into Cancer and Nutrition-Norfolk prospective study. Am Heart J. 2011;162(2):246-5

[141] Gurven M, Kaplan H, Winking J, Eid Rodriguez D, Vasunilashorn S, Kim JK, Finch C, Crimmins E. Inflammation and infection do not promote arterial aging and cardiovascular disease risk factors among lean horticulturalists. PLoS One. 2009;4(8):e6590.

[142] www westonprice org

[143] DrogeW. Oxidative stress and ageing: is ageing a cysteine deficiency syndrome? Philos Trans R Soc Lond B Biol Sci. 2005;360(1464):2355-72.

[144] Factor VM, Laskowska D, Jensen MR, Woitach JT, Popescu NC, Thorgeirsson SS. Vitamin E reduces chromosomal damage and inhibits hepatic tumor formation in a transgenic mouse model. Proc Natl Acad Sci U S A. 2000;97(5):2196-201.

[145] Singh I, Turner AH, Sinclair AJ, Li D, Hawley JA. Effects of gamma-tocopherol supplementation on thrombotic risk factors. Asia Pac J Clin Nutr. 2007;16(3):422-8.

[146] Hamidi MS, Corey PN, Cheung AM. Effects of vitamin E on bone turnover markers among US postmenopausal women. J Bone Miner Res. 2012;27(6):1368-80.

[147] Sinha R, Patterson BH, Mangels AR, Levander OA, Gibson T, Taylor PR, Block G. Determinants of plasma vitamin E in healthy males. Cancer Epidemiol Biomarkers Prev. 1993;2(5):473-9.

[148] National Center for Health Statistics. Mortality Report. Hyattsville, MD: U.S. Department of Health and Human Services; 2002.

[149] US Department of Health and Human Services, National Center for Health Statistics. Health, United States, 2010: With Special Feature on Death and Dying. Hyattsville, MD. 2011. Table 94: Prescription Drug Use In The Last Month, page 318, Trend Tables.

[150] Downs JR, Clearfield M, Weis S, Whitney E et al. Primary prevention of acute coronary events with lovastatin in men and women with average cholesterol levels: results of AFCAPS/TexCAPS. Air Force/Texas Coronary Atherosclerosis Prevention Study. JAMA. 1998;279(20):1615-22.

[151] Bengmark S. Advanced glycation and lipoxidation end products--amplifiers of inflammation: the role of food. JPEN J Parenter Enteral Nutr. 2007;31(5):430-40.

[152] Gil A, Bengmark S. Advanced glycation and lipoxidation end products--amplifiers of inflammation: the role of food. Nutr Hosp. 2007;22(6):625-40.

[153] The Sharp Brains Guide to Brain Fitness: 18 Interviews with Scientists, Practical Advice, and Product Reviews, To Keep Your Brain Sharp. Alvaro Fernandez & Elkhonon Goldberg.

[154] Relaxation Revolution: Enhancing Your Personal Health Through the Science and Genetics of Mind Body Healing. H. Benson, MD.

[155] Bourre JM. Effects of nutrients (in food) on the structure and function of the nervous system: update on dietary requirements for brain. Part 1: micronutrients. J Nutr Health Aging. 2006:377-85.

[156] Schaefer EJ, Bongard V, Beiser AS, Lamon-Fava S, Robins SJ, Au R, Tucker KL, Kyle DJ, Wilson PW, Wolf PA. Plasma phosphatidylcholine docosahexaenoic acid content and risk of dementia and Alzheimer disease: the Framingham Heart Study. Arch Neurol. 2006;63(11):1545-50.

[157] Hibbeln JR, Nieminen LR, Blasbalg TL, Riggs JA, Lands WE. Healthy intakes of n-3 and n-6 fatty acids: estimations considering worldwide diversity. Am J Clin Nutr. 2006 Jun (6 Suppl):1483S-1493S.

[158] Circulation. 2002; 106: 2747-57. AHA Scientific Statement Fish Consumption, Fish Oil, Omega-3 Fatty Acids, and Cardiovascular Disease. TABLE 5. Summary of Recommendations for Omega-3 Fatty Acid Intake:

[159] Dietary supplementation with n-3 polyunsaturated fatty acids and vitamin E after myocardial infarction: results of the GISSI-Prevenzione trial. Gruppo Italiano per lo Studio della Sopravvivenza nell'Infarto miocardico. Lancet. 1999;354(9177):447-55.

[160] Gerster H. Can adults adequately convert alpha-linolenic acid (18:3n-3) to eicosapentaenoic acid (20:5n-3) and docosahexaenoic acid (22:6n-3)? Int J Vitam Nutr Res. 1998;68(3):159-73.

[161] Johnson EJ, Schaefer EJ. Potential role of dietary n-3 fatty acids in the prevention of dementia and macular degeneration. Am J Clin Nutr. 2006;83(6 Suppl):1494S-1498S.

[162] Calabrese V, Cornelius C, Mancuso C, Lentile R, Stella AM, Butterfield DA. Redox homeostasis and cellular stress response in aging and neurodegeneration. Methods Mol Biol. 2010;610:285-308.

163 Debette S, Beiser A, Hoffmann U, Decarli C, O'Donnell CJ, Massaro JM, Au R et al. Visceral fat is associated with lower brain volume in healthy middle-aged adults. Ann Neurol. 2010;68(2):136-44.
164 Kawahara M, Kuroda Y. Molecular mechanism of neurodegeneration induced by Alzheimer's beta-amyloid protein: channel formation and disruption of calcium homeostasis. Brain Res Bull. 2000;53(4):389-97.
165 Kawahara M, Kuroda Y. Intracellular calcium changes in neuronal cells induced by Alzheimer's beta-amyloid protein are blocked by estradiol and cholesterol. Cell Mol Neurobiol. 2001;21(1):1-13.
166 Potempa LA, Kubak BM, Gewurz H. Effect of divalent metal ions and pH upon the binding reactivity of human serum amyloid P component, a C-reactive protein homologue, for zymosan. Preferential reactivity in the presence of copper and acidic pH. J Biol Chem. 1985;260(22):12142-7.
167 Tan ZS, Beiser AS, Fox CS, Au R, Himali JJ, Debette S, et al. Association of metabolic dysregulation with volumetric brain magnetic resonance imaging and cognitive markers of subclinical brain aging in middle-aged adults: the Framingham Offspring Study. Diabetes Care. 2011;34(8):1766-70.
168 Scarmeas N, Luchsinger JA, Schupf N, Brickman AM, Cosentino S, Tang MX, Stern Y. Physical Activity, Diet, and Risk of Alzheimer Disease. JAMA 2009; 302(6): 627-37.
169 Krikorian R, Shidler MD, Nash TA, Kalt W, Vinqvist-Tymchuk MR, Shukitt-Hale B et al. Blueberry supplementation improves memory in older adults. J Agric Food Chem. 2010;58(7):3996-4000.
170 Joseph JA, Shukitt-Hale B, Willis LM. Grape juice, berries, and walnuts affect brain aging and behavior. J Nutr. 2009;139(9):1813S-7S.
171 Rayssiguier Y, Durlach J, Gueux E, Rock E, Mazur A. Magnesium and ageing. I. Experimental data: importance of oxidative damage. Magnes Res. 1993;6(4):369-78.
172 Wallwork JC. Zinc and the central nervous system. Prog Food Nutr Sci. 1987;11(2):203-47.
173 Naurath HJ, Joosten E, Riezler R, Stabler SP, Allen RH, Lindenbaum J. Effects of vitamin B12, folate, and vitamin B6 supplements in elderly people with normal serum vitamin concentrations. Lancet. 1995;346(8967):85-9.
174 McCaddon A, Hudson P, Ellis D, Hill D, Lloyd A. Correspondance. Lancet 2002; 360 (9327):173
175 Smith AD, Smith SM, de Jager CA, Whitbread P, Johnston C, Agacinski G, Oulhaj A, Bradley KM, Jacoby R, Refsum H. Homocysteine-lowering by B vitamins slows the rate of accelerated brain atrophy in mild cognitive impairment: a randomized controlled trial. PLoS One. 2010;5(9):e12244.
176 Marcuard SP, Albernaz L, Khazanie PG. Omeprazole therapy causes malabsorption of cyanocobalamin (vitamin B12) Ann Intern Med. 1994;120(3):211-5.
177 Knox TA, Spiegelman D, Skinner SC, Gorbach S. Diarrhea and abnormalities of gastrointestinal function in a cohort of men and women with HIV infection. Am J Gastroenterol. 2000;95(12):3482-9.

178 Woods MN, Tang AM, Forrester J, Jones C, Hendricks K, Ding B, Knox TA. Effect of dietary intake and protease inhibitors on serum vitamin B12 levels in a cohort of human immunodeficiency virus-positive patients. Clin Infect Dis. 2003;37 Suppl 2:S124-31.
179 Möller HJ. Relativising the significance of the results of metaanalyses: comments on the metaanalysis by Kirsch et al. 2008 regarding the effectiveness of modern antidepressants. MMW Fortschr Med. 2009;151(13):80-3.
180 Das UN. Folic acid and polyunsaturated fatty acids improve cognitive function and prevent depression, dementia, and Alzheimer's disease--but how and why? Prostaglandins Leukot Essent Fatty Acids. 2008;78(1):11-9.
181 Catena-Dell'Osso M, Bellantuono C, Consoli G, Baroni S, Rotella F et al. Inflammatory and neurodegenerative pathways in depression: a new avenue for antidepressant development? Curr Med Chem. 2011;18(2):245-55.
182 Maes M, Yirmyia R, Noraberg J, Brene S, Hibbeln J, Perini G, Kubera M, Bob P, Lerer B, Maj M. The inflammatory & neurodegenerative (I&ND) hypothesis of depression: leads for future research and new drug developments in depression. Metab Brain Dis. 2009; 24(1):27-53.
183 James Gordon, MD. *Unstuck: Your Guide to the Seven-Stage Journey Out of Depression* by James S. Gordon (2009) Pengiun Group, New York.
184 Henry Emmons, MD. *The Chemistry of Calm: A Powerful, Drug-Free Plan to Quiet Your Fears and Overcome Your Anxiety.* 2010. Touchstone Books/Simon & Schuster; New York.
185 Steegmans PH, Hoes AW, Bak AA, van der Does E et al. Higher prevalence of depressive symptoms in middle-aged men with low serum cholesterol levels. Psychosom Med. 2000;62(2):205-11.
186 Greenblatt J. *The Breakthrough Depression Solution: A Personalized 9-Step Method for Beathing The Physical Causes of Your Depression.* Sunrise River Press. ISBN 978-1-934716-15-1
187 Dressman J, Kincer J, Matveev SV, Guo L, Greenberg RN, Guerin T, Meade D, Li XA, Zhu W, Uittenbogaard A, Wilson ME, Smart EJ. HIV protease inhibitors promote atherosclerotic lesion formation independent of dyslipidemia by increasing CD36-dependent cholesteryl ester accumulation in macrophages. J Clin Invest. 2003;111(3):389-97.
188 Bradshaw EL, Li XA, Guerin T, Everson WV, Wilson ME, Bruce-Keller AJ, Greenberg RN, Guo L, Ross SA, Smart EJ. Nucleoside reverse transcriptase inhibitors prevent HIV protease inhibitor-induced atherosclerosis by ubiquitination and degradation of protein kinase C. Am J Physiol Cell Physiol. 2006;291(6):C1271-8.
189 Lippi G, Franchini M, Favaloro EJ, Targher G. Moderate red wine consumption and cardiovascular disease risk: beyond the "French paradox". Semin Thromb Hemost. 2010;36(1):59-70.
190 Liu S, Manson JE, Lee IM, Cole SR, Hennekens CH, Willett WC, Buring JE.
Fruit and vegetable intake and risk of cardiovascular disease: the Women's Health Study. Am J Clin Nutr. 2000 Oct;72(4):922-8.
191 Richard A. Kronmal, PhD; Kevin C. Cain, PhD; Zhan Ye, MD; Gilbert S. Omenn, MD, PhD. Total Serum Cholesterol Levels and Mortality Risk as a Function of Age. A Report Based on the Framingham Data. *Arch Intern Med.* 1993;153(9):1065-1073.
192 Find link to the letter at: http://www.cas.usf.edu/news/s/176 .
193 Schatz IJ, Masaki K, Yano K, Chen R, Rodriguez BL, Curb JD. Cholesterol and all-cause mortality in elderly people from the Honolulu Heart Program: a cohort study. Lancet. 2001;358(9279):351-5.

[194] Mozaffarian D. Effects of dietary fats versus carbohydrates on coronary heart disease: a review of the evidence. Curr Atheroscler Rep. 2005;7(6):435-45.

[195] Mozaffarian D. The great fat debate: taking the focus off of saturated fat. J Am Diet Assoc. 2011;111(5):665-6.

[196] http://mycourses.med.harvard.edu/MediaPlayer/Player.aspx?v={FD6EDE1D-759F-4D31-A162-E3767C12155B} Mozaffarian Harvard Lecture.

[197] Simopoulos AP. Evolutionary aspects of omega-3 fatty acids in the food supply. Prostaglandins Leukot Essent Fatty Acids. 1999;60(5-6):421-9.

[198] de Lorgeril M, Salen P, Martin JL, Monjaud I, Delaye J, Mamelle N. Mediterranean diet, traditional risk factors, and the rate of cardiovascular complications after myocardial infarction: final report of the Lyon Diet Heart Study. Circulation. 1999;99(6):779-85.

[199] Joshipura KJ, Hu FB, Manson JE, Stampfer MJ, Rimm EB, Speizer FE, Colditz G, Ascherio A, Rosner B, Spiegelman D, Willett WC. The Effect of Fruit and Vegetable Intake on Risk for Coronary Heart Disease. Ann Intern Med. 2001;134:1106-1114.

[200] Kannel WB. Cholesterol and risk of coronary heart disease and mortality in men. Clin Chem. 1988;34(8B):B53-9.

[201] Abramson, John. Overdosed America, The Broken Promise of American Medicine.

[202] Corti MC, Guralnik JM, Salive ME, Harris T, Field TS, Wallace RB, Berkman LF et al. HDL cholesterol predicts coronary heart disease mortality in older persons. JAMA. 1995;274(7):539-44.

[203] Hausenloy DJ, Yellon DM. Targeting residual cardiovascular risk: raising high-density lipoprotein cholesterol levels. Heart. 2008;94(6):706-14.

[204] Murata H, Hruz PW, Mueckler M. The mechanism of insulin resistance caused by HIV protease inhibitor therapy. J Biol Chem. 2000;275(27):20251-4.

[205] Monroe AK, Dobs AS, Xu X, Palella FJ, Kingsley LA et al. Sex hormones, insulin resistance, and diabetes mellitus among men with or at risk for HIV infection. JAIDS 2011;58(2):173-80.

[206] Salazar J, Guardiola M, Ferré R, Coll B, Alonso-Villaverde C et al. Association of a polymorphism in the promoter of the cellular retinoic acid-binding protein II gene (CRABP2) with increased circulating low-density lipoprotein cholesterol. Clin Chem Lab Med. 2007;45(5):615-20.

[207] Crowe SM, Westhorpe CL, Mukhamedova N, Jaworowski A, Sviridov D et al. The macrophage: the intersection between HIV infection and atherosclerosis. J Leukoc Biol. 2010;87(4):589-98.

[208] Mondal D, Pradhan L, Ali M, Agrawal KC. HAART drugs induce oxidative stress in human endothelial cells and increase endothelial recruitment of mononuclear cells: exacerbation by inflammatory cytokines and amelioration by antioxidants. Cardiovasc Toxicol. 2004;4(3):287-302.

[209] Simopoulos AP. Evolutionary aspects of omega-3 fatty acids in the food supply. Prostaglandins Leukot Essent Fatty Acids. 1999; 60(5-6): 421-9.

[210] Stampfer MJ, Hennekens CH, Manson JE, Colditz GA, Rosner B, Willett WC. Vitamin E consumption and the risk of coronary disease in women. N Engl J Med. 1993;328(20):1444-9.

[211] Lee IM, Cook NR, Gaziano JM, Gordon D, Ridker PM, Manson JE, Hennekens CH, Buring JE. Vitamin E in the primary prevention of cardiovascular disease and cancer: the Women's Health Study: a randomized controlled trial. JAMA. 2005;294(1):56-65.

[212] Stephens NG, Parsons A, Schofield PM, Kelly F, Cheeseman K, Mitchinson MJ. Randomised controlled trial of vitamin E in patients with coronary disease: Cambridge Heart Antioxidant Study (CHAOS). Lancet. 1996;347(9004):781-6.

[213] Gutierrez AD, de Serna DG, Robinson I, Schade DS. The response of gamma vitamin E to varying dosages of alpha vitamin E plus vitamin C. Metabolism. 2009;58(4):469-78.

[214] Gutierrez AD, de Serna DG, Robinson I, Schade DS. The response of gamma vitamin E to varying dosages of alpha vitamin E plus vitamin C. Metabolism. 2009;58(4):469-78.

[215] Brown TT, Tassiopoulos K, Bosch RJ, Shikuma C, McComsey GA. Association between systemic inflammation and incident diabetes in HIV-infected patients after initiation of antiretroviral therapy. Diabetes Care. 2010;33(10):2244-9.

[216] Kenneth Lichtenstein, R Debes, K Wood, S Bozzette, K Buchacz, J Brooks, and HIV Outpatient Study Investigators. Statin Use Is Associated with Incident Diabetes Mellitus among Patients in the HIV Outpatient Study. Paper #767; CROI 2013, Atlanta, GA, USA March 3-6, 2013

[217] Aukrust P, Müller F, Svardal AM, Ueland T, Berge RK, Frøland SS. Disturbed glutathione metabolism and decreased antioxidant levels in human immunodeficiency virus-infected patients during highly active antiretroviral therapy--potential immunomodulatory effects of antioxidants. J Infect Dis. 2003;188(2):232-8.

[218] Birjmohun RS, Hutten BA, Kastelein JJ, Stroes ES. Increasing HDL cholesterol with extended-release nicotinic acid: from promise to practice. Neth J Med. 2004;62(7):229-34.

[219] Canner PL, Berge KG, Wenger NK, Stamler J, Friedman L, Prineas RJ et al. Fifteen year mortality in Coronary Drug Project patients: long-term benefit with niacin. J Am Coll Cardiol. 1986;8(6):1245-55.

[220] Kamanna VS, Kashyap ML. Mechanism of action of niacin. Am J Cardiol. 2008;101(8A):20B-26B.

[221] Chapman MJ, Assmann G, Fruchart JC, Shepherd J, Sirtori C; European Consensus Panel on HDL-C. Raising high-density lipoprotein cholesterol with reduction of cardiovascular risk: the role of nicotinic acid--a position paper developed by the European Consensus Panel on HDL-C. Curr Med Res Opin. 2004;20(8):1253-68.

[222] Kinscherf R, Cafaltzis K, Röder F, Hildebrandt W, Edler L, Deigner HP, Breitkreutz R, Feussner G, Kreuzer J, Werle E, Michel G, Metz J, Dröge W. Cholesterol levels linked to abnormal plasma thiol concentrations and thiol/disulfide redox status in hyperlipidemic subjects. Free Radic Biol Med. 2003;35(10):1286-92.

[223] Dröge W. Cysteine and glutathione deficiency in AIDS patients: a rationale for the treatment with N-acetyl-cysteine. Pharmacology. 1993;46(2):61-5.

[224] Breitkreutz R, Holm S, Pittack N, Beichert M, Babylon A, Yodoi J, Dröge W. Massive loss of sulfur in HIV infection. AIDS Res Hum Retroviruses. 2000;16(3):203-9.

[225] Breitkreutz R, Pittack N, Nebe CT, Schuster D, Brust J, Beichert M, Hack V, Daniel V, Edler L, Dröge W. Improvement of immune functions in HIV infection by sulfur supplementation: two randomized trials. J Mol Med (Berl). 2000;78(1):55-62.

[226] Franceschini G, Werba JP, Safa O, Gikalov I, Sirtori CR. Dose-related increase of HDL-cholesterol levels after N-acetylcysteine in man. Pharmacol Res. 1993;28(3):213-8.

[227] Li JZ, Chen ML, Wang S, Dong J, Zeng P, Hou LW. Apparent protective effect of high density lipoprotein against coronary heart disease in the elderly. Chin Med J (Engl). 2004;117(4):511-5.

[228] Jones DP, Mody VC Jr, Carlson JL, Lynn MJ, Sternberg P Jr. Redox analysis of human plasma allows separation of pro-oxidant events of aging from decline in antioxidant defenses. Free Radic Biol Med. 2002;33(9):1290-300.

[229] Ruiz Fuentes MC, Moreno Ayuso JM, Ruiz Fuentes N, Vargas Palomares JF, Asensio Peinado C, Osuna Ortega A. Treatment with N-acetylcysteine in stable renal transplantation. Transplant Proc. 2008;40(9):2897-9.

[230] Herzenberg LA, De Rosa SC, Dubs JG, Roederer M, Anderson MT, Ela SW, Deresinski SC, Herzenberg LA. Glutathione deficiency is associated with impaired survival in HIV disease. Proc Natl Acad Sci U S A. 1997;94(5):1967-72.

[231] Kalebic T, Kinter A, Poli G, Anderson ME, Meister A, Fauci AS. Suppression of human immunodeficiency virus expression in chronically infected monocytic cells by glutathione, glutathione ester, and N-acetylcysteine. Proc Natl Acad Sci U S A. 1991;88(3):986-90.

[232] Micha R, Mozaffarian D. Saturated fat and cardiometabolic risk factors, coronary heart disease, stroke, and diabetes: a fresh look at the evidence. Lipids. 2010;45(10):893-905.

[233] Huang CB, Alimova Y, Myers TM, Ebersole JL. Short- and medium-chain fatty acids exhibit antimicrobial activity for oral microorganisms. Arch Oral Biol. 2011;56(7):650-4.

[234] Nakatsuji T, Kao MC, Fang JY, Zouboulis CC, Zhang L, Gallo RL, Huang CM. Antimicrobial property of lauric acid against Propionibacterium acnes: its therapeutic potential for inflammatory acne vulgaris. J Invest Dermatol. 2009;129(10):2480-8. doi: 10.1038/jid.2009.93.

[235] Yao J, Chen S, Mao Z, Cadenas E, Brinton RD. 2-Deoxy-D-glucose treatment induces ketogenesis, sustains mitochondrial function, and reduces pathology in female mouse model of Alzheimer's disease. PLoS One. 2011;6(7):e21788.

[236] Newport, Mary T. Alzheimer's Disease: What If There Was a Cure?: The Story of Ketones. Publisher: Basic Health Publications. ISBN: 1591202930

[237] Kapoor R, Huang YS. Gamma linolenic acid: an antiinflammatory omega-6 fatty acid. Curr Pharm Biotechnol. 2006;7(6):531-4.

[238] Horrobin DF, Manku MS. How do polyunsaturated fatty acids lower plasma cholesterol levels? Lipids. 1983;18(8):558-62.

[239] Kröger J, Schulze MB. Recent insights into the relation of Δ5 desaturase and Δ6 desaturase activity to the development of type 2 diabetes. Curr Opin Lipidol. 2012;23(1):4-10.

[240] Horrobin DF. Fatty acid metabolism in health and disease: the role of delta-6-desaturase. Am J Clin Nutr. 1993;57(5 Suppl):732S-736S.

[241] Albert CM, Hennekens CH, O'Donnell CJ, Ajani UA, Carey VJ, Willett WC, Ruskin JN, Manson JE. Fish consumption and risk of sudden cardiac death. JAMA. 1998;279(1):23-8.

[242] Dietary supplementation with n-3 polyunsaturated fatty acids and vitamin E after myocardial infarction: results of the GISSI-Prevenzione trial. Gruppo Italiano per lo Studio della Sopravvivenza nell'Infarto miocardico. Lancet. 1999;354(9177):447-55.

[243] Woods MN, Wanke CA, Ling PR, Hendricks KM, Tang AM, Knox TA, Andersson CE, Dong KR, Skinner SC, Bistrian BR. Effect of a dietary intervention and n-3 fatty acid supplementation on measures of serum lipid and insulin sensitivity in persons with HIV. Am J Clin Nutr. 2009;90(6):1566-78.

[244] Christensen JH. n-3 fatty acids and the risk of sudden cardiac death. Emphasis on heart rate variability. Dan Med Bull. 2003;50(4):347-67.

[245] Das UN. Essential fatty acids and their metabolites could function as endogenous HMG-CoA reductase and ACE enzyme inhibitors, anti-arrhythmic, anti-hypertensive, anti-atherosclerotic, anti-inflammatory, cytoprotective, and cardioprotective molecules. Lipids Health Dis. 2008;7:37.

[246] Dobryniewski J, Szajda SD, Waszkiewicz N, Zwierz K. [The gamma-linolenic acid (GLA)--the therapeutic value]. Przegl Lek. 2007;64(2):100-2.

[247] Horrobin DF. Essential fatty acids in the management of impaired nerve function in diabetes. Diabetes. 1997; 46 Suppl 2:S90-93.

[248] Tremblay AJ, Després JP, Piché ME, Nadeau A, Bergeron J, Alméras N, Tremblay A, Lemieux S. Associations between the fatty acid content of triglyceride, visceral adipose tissue accumulation, and components of the insulin resistance syndrome. Metabolism. 2004 Mar;53(3):310-7.

[249] Levy E, Thibault L, Garofalo C, Messier M, Lepage G, Ronco N, Roy CC. Combined (n-3 and n-6) essential fatty deficiency is a potent modulator of plasma lipids, lipoprotein composition, and lipolytic enzymes. J Lipid Res. 1990;31(11):2009-17.

[250] Hadigan C, Liebau J, Torriani M, Andersen R, Grinspoon S. Improved triglycerides and insulin sensitivity with 3 months of acipimox in human immunodeficiency virus-infected patients with hypertriglyceridemia. J Clin Endocrinol Metab. 2006;91(11):4438-44.

[251] Guo W, Wong S, Pudney J, Jasuja R, Hua N, Jiang L, Miller A, Hruz PW, Hamilton JA, Bhasin S. Acipimox, an inhibitor of lipolysis, attenuates atherogenesis in LDLR-null mice treated with HIV protease inhibitor ritonavir. Arterioscler Thromb Vasc Biol. 2009;29(12):2028-32.

[252] Miller TL, Wolin MJ. Pathways of Acetate, Propionate, and Butyrate Formation by the Human Fecal Microbial Flora. Applied and Environmental Microbiology; 62(5):1589–1592.

[253] Kallio P, Kolehmainen M, Laaksonen DE, Kekäläinen J, Salopuro T, Sivenius K, Pulkkinen L, Mykkänen HM, Niskanen L, Uusitupa M, Poutanen KS. Dietary carbohydrate modification induces alterations in gene expression in abdominal subcutaneous adipose tissue in persons with the metabolic syndrome: the FUNGENUT Study. Am J Clin Nutr. 2007;85(5):1417-27.

[254] Allan CB, Lutz W. Life Without Bread; how a low-carb diet can save your life. 2000 McGraw-Hill. New York.

[255] DasUN. Essential fatty acids and their metabolites could function as endogenous HMG-CoA reductase and ACE enzyme inhibitors, anti-arrhythmic, anti-hypertensive, anti-atherosclerotic, anti-inflammatory, cytoprotective, and cardioprotective molecules. Lipids Health Dis. 2008;7:37.

[256] Levy E, Thibault L, Garofalo C, Messier M, Lepage G, Ronco N, Roy CC. Combined (n-3 and n-6) essential fatty deficiency is a potent modulator of plasma lipids, lipoprotein composition, and lipolytic enzymes. J Lipid Res. 1990; 31(11):2009-17.

[257] Damasceno NR, Pérez-Heras A, Serra M, Cofán M, Sala-Vila A, Salas-Salvadó J, Ros E. Crossover study of diets enriched with virgin olive oil, walnuts or almonds. Effects on lipids and other cardiovascular risk markers. Nutr Metab Cardiovasc Dis. 2011;21 Suppl 1:S14-20.

[258] Li SC, Liu YH, Liu JF, Chang WH, Chen CM, Chen CY. Almond consumption improved glycemic control and lipid profiles in patients with type 2 diabetes mellitus. Metabolism. 2011;60(4):474-9.

[259] Ros E, Núñez I, Pérez-Heras A, Serra M et al. A walnut diet improves endothelial function in hypercholesterolemic subjects: a randomized crossover trial. Circulation. 2004;109(13):1609-14.

[260] Wilson PW, D'Agostino RB, Levy D, Belanger AM, Silbershatz H, Kannel WB. Prediction of coronary heart disease using risk factor categories. Circulation. 1998;97(18):1837-47.

[261] http://www.framinghamheartstudy.org/risk/hrdcoronary.html

[262] Burdo TH, Lo J, Abbara S, Wei J, DeLelys ME, Preffer F, Rosenberg ES, Williams KC, Grinspoon S. Soluble CD163, a novel marker of activated macrophages, is elevated and associated with noncalcified coronary plaque in HIV-infected patients. J Infect Dis. 2011;204(8):1227-36.

[263] d'Ettorre G, Paiardini M, Zaffiri L, Andreotti M, Ceccarelli G, Rizza C, Indinnimeo M, Vella S, Mastroianni CM, Silvestri G, Vullo V. HIV persistence in the gut mucosa of HIV-infected subjects undergoing antiretroviral therapy correlates with immune activation and increased levels of LPS. Curr HIV Res. 2011;9(3):148-53.

[264] Hamilton SJ, Chew GT, Watts GF. Coenzyme Q10 improves endothelial dysfunction in statin-treated type 2 diabetic patients. Diabetes Care. 2009; 32(5):810-2.

[265] Chester JG, Rudolph JL. Vital signs in older patients: age-related changes. J Am Med Dir Assoc. 2011;12(5):337-43.

[266] Cotugna N, Wolpert S. Sodium recommendations for special populations and the resulting implications. J Community Health. 2011;36(5):874-82.

[267] Sacks FM, Appel LJ, Moore TJ, Obarzanek E, Vollmer WM, Svetkey LP, Bray GA, Vogt TM, Cutler JA, Windhauser MM, Lin PH, Karanja N. A dietary approach to prevent hypertension: a review of the Dietary Approaches to Stop Hypertension (DASH) Study. Clin Cardiol. 1999;22(7 Suppl):III6-10.

[268] Moore R, Webb G. The K Factor: Reversing and Preventing High Blood Pressure Without Drugs. 1996 MacMillan Publ.

[269] Luther JM, Brown NJ. The renin-angiotensin-aldosterone system and glucose homeostasis. Trends Pharmacol Sci. 2011;32(12):734-9.

[270] Littaru GP, Ho L, Folkers K. Deficiency of coenzyme Q 10 in human heart disease. I. Int J Vitam Nutr Res. 1972;42(2):291-305.

[271] Gadaleta MN, Cormio A, Pesce V, Lezza AM, Cantatore P. Aging and mitochondria. Biochimie. 1998;80(10):863-70.

[272] Linnane AW, Kovalenko S, Gingold EB: The universality of bioenergetic disease: age associated cellular bioenergetic degradation and amelioration therapy. Ann NY Acad Sci, 1998; 854: 202-213.

[273] Folkers K, Langsjoen P, Willis R, Richardson P, Xia L-J, Ye C-Q, Tamagawa H: Lovastatin decreases coenzyme Q levels in humans. Proc Natl Acad Sci USA, 1990; 87: 8931-8934.

[274] Mortensen SA. Perspectives on Therpay of cardiovascular diseases with coenzyme Q10 (ubiquinone). Clin Investig. 1993;71(8 Suppl):S116-23.

[275] Rusciani L, Proietti I, Rusciani A, Paradisi A et al. Low plasma coenzyme Q10 levels as an independent prognostic factor for melanoma progression. J Am Acad Dermatol. 2006;54(2):234-41.

[276] Lockwood K., Moesgaard S., Yamamoto T., Folkers K. Progress on therapy of breast cancer with vitamin Q10 and the regression of metastases. Biochem Biophys Res Commun.1995 ;212(1):172-7.

[277] Rudnicka D, Oszmiana A, Finch DK, Strickland I, Schofield DJ, Lowe DC, Sleeman MA, Davis DM. Rituximab causes a polarisation of B cells which augments its therapeutic function in NK cell-mediated antibody-dependent cellular cytotoxicity. Blood. 2013 Apr 23. [Epub ahead of print]

[278] Lee JH, Jarreau T, Prasad A, Lavie C, O'Keefe J, Ventura H. Nutritional assessment in heart failure patients. Congest Heat Fail. 2011; 17(4):199-203

[279] Sole MJ, Jeejeebhoy KN. Conditioned nutritional requirements: therapeutic relevance to heart failure. Herz. 2002; 27(2):174-8.

[280] Keith ME, Walsh NA, Darling PB, Hanninen SA, Thirugnanam S, Leong-Poi H, Barr A, Sole MJ. B-vitamin deficiency in hospitalized patients with heart failure. J Am Diet Assoc. 2009;109(8):1406-10.

[281] Parcell S. Sulfur in human nutrition and applications in medicine. Altern Med Rev. 2002;7(1):22-44.

[282] Langsjoen H, Langsjoen P, Langsjoen P, Willis R, Folkers K. Usefulness of coenzyme Q10 in clinical cardiology: a long-term study. Mol Aspects Med. 1994;15 Suppl:s165-75.

[283] Shahzad K, Chokshi A, Schulze PC. Supplementation of glutamine and omega-3 polyunsaturated Fatty acids as a novel therapeutic intervention targeting metabolic dysfunction and exercise intolerance in patients with heart failure. Curr Clin Pharmacol. 2011;6(4):288-94.

[284] Rizos I. Three-year survival of patients with heart failure caused by dilated cardiomyopathy and L-carnitine administration. Am Heart J. 2000;139(2 Pt 3):S120-123.

[285] Grassi M, Petraccia L, Mennuni G, Fontana M, Scarno A, Sabetta S, Fraioli A. Changes, functional disorders and diseases in the gastrointestinal tract of elderly. Nutr Hosp. 2011;26(4):659-68.

[286] Talley NJ, Fleming KC, Evans JM, O'Keefe EA, Weaver AL, Zinsmeister AR, Melton LJ 3rd. Constipation in an elderly community: a study of prevalence and potential risk factors. Am J Gastroenterol. 1996;91(1):19-25.

[287] Kumar V, Sinha AK, Makkar HP, de Boeck G, Becker K. Dietary roles of non-starch polysachharides in human nutrition: a review. Crit Rev Food Sci Nutr. 2012;52(10):899-935.

[288] Musso G, Gambino R, Cassader M. Obesity, diabetes, and gut microbiota: the hygiene hypothesis expanded? Diabetes Care. 2010;33(10):2277-84.

[289] Nilsson AC, Östman EM, Knudsen KE, Holst JJ, Björck IM. A cereal-based evening meal rich in indigestible carbohydrates increases plasma butyrate the next morning. J Nutr. 2010;140(11):1932-6.

[290] Abou-Donia MB, El-Masry EM, Abdel-Rahman AA, McLendon RE, Schiffman SS. Splenda alters gut microflora and increases intestinal p-glycoprotein and cytochrome p-450 in male rats. J Toxicol Environ Health A. 2008;71(21):1415-29.

[291] Purohit V, Bode JC, Bode C, Brenner DA, Choudhry MA, Hamilton F, Kang YJ, Keshavarzian A, Rao R, Sartor RB, Swanson C, Turner JR. Alcohol, intestinal bacterial growth, intestinal permeability to endotoxin, and medical consequences: summary of a symposium. Alcohol. 2008;42(5):349-61.

[292] Shindo K, Machida M, Fukumura M, Koide K, Yamazaki R. Omeprazole induces altered bile acid metabolism. Gut. 1998;42(2):266-71.

[293] Eom CS, Jeon CY, Lim JW, Cho EG, Park SM, Lee KS. Use of acid-suppressive drugs and risk of pneumonia: a systematic review and meta-analysis. CMAJ. 2011;183(3):310-9.

[294] Del Piano M, Carmagnola S, Anderloni A, Andorno S, Ballarè M, Balzarini M, Montino F, Orsello M, Pagliarulo M, Sartori M, Tari R, Sforza F, Capurso L. The use of probiotics in healthy volunteers with evacuation disorders and hard stools: a double-blind, randomized, placebo-controlled study. J Clin Gastroenterol. 2010;44 Suppl 1:S30-4.

[295] Judy Shabert, MD, MPH, RD Glutamine, The Ultimate Nutrient, 1994. Avery

[296] Bradford GS, Taylor CT. Omeprazole and vitamin B12 deficiency. Ann Pharmacother. 1999;33(5):641-3.

[297] Mazziotti G, Canalis E, Giustina A. Drug-induced osteoporosis: mechanisms and clinical implications. Am J Med. 2010;123(10):877-84.

[298] Kallio P, Kolehmainen M, Laaksonen DE, Kekäläinen J, Salopuro T, Sivenius K, Pulkkinen L, Mykkänen HM, Niskanen L, Uusitupa M, Poutanen KS. Dietary carbohydrate modification induces alterations in gene expression in abdominal subcutaneous adipose tissue in persons with the metabolic syndrome: the FUNGENUT Study. Am J Clin Nutr. 2007;85(5):1417-27.

[299] Gordon SN, Cervasi B, Odorizzi P, Silverman R, Aberra F, Ginsberg G, Estes JD, Paiardini M, Frank I, Silvestri G. Disruption of intestinal CD4+ T cell homeostasis is a key marker of systemic CD4+ T cell activation in HIV-infected individuals. J Immunol. 2010;185(9):5169-79.

[300] Estes J, Baker JV, Brenchley JM, Khoruts A, Barthold JL, Bantle A, Reilly CS, Beilman GJ, George ME, Douek DC, Haase AT, Schacker TW. Collagen deposition limits immune reconstitution in the gut. J Infect Dis. 2008;198(4):456-64.

[301] Merlini E, Bai F, Bellistrì GM, Tincati C, d'Arminio Monforte A, Marchetti G. Evidence for polymicrobic flora translocating in peripheral blood of HIV-infected patients with poor immune response to antiretroviral therapy. PLoS One. 2011;6(4):e18580.

[302] d'Ettorre G, Paiardini M, Zaffiri L, Andreotti M, Ceccarelli G, Rizza C, Indinnimeo M, Vella S, Mastroianni CM, Silvestri G, Vullo V. HIV persistence in the gut mucosa of HIV-infected subjects undergoing antiretroviral therapy correlates with immune activation and increased levels of LPS. Curr HIV Res. 2011;9(3):148-53.

[303] Marks MA, Rabkin CS, Engels EA, Busch E, Kopp W, Rager H, Goedert JJ, Chaturvedi AK. Markers of microbial translocation and risk of AIDS-related lymphoma. AIDS. 2013: 27(3):469-74.

[304] Stebbing J, Gazzard B, Mandalia S, Teague A, Waterston A, Marvin V, Nelson M, Bower M. Antiretroviral treatment regimens and immune parameters in the prevention of systemic AIDS-related non-Hodgkin's lymphoma. J Clin Oncol. 2004;22(11):2177-83.

[305] Karinch AM, Pan M, Lin CM, Strange R, Souba WW. Glutamine metabolism in sepsis and infection. J Nutr. 2001;131(9 Suppl):2535S-8S; discussion 2550S-1S.

[306] Aosasa S, Wells-Byrum D, Alexander JW, Ogle CK. Influence of glutamine-supplemented Caco-2 cells on cytokine production of mononuclear cells. JPEN J Parenter Enteral Nutr. 2003;27(5):333-9.

[307] Jing K, Sun M. [Relationship between the regulation of intestinal NF-κB and TNF-α by glutamine and the protective effects of glutamine against intestinal injury]. Zhongguo Dang Dai Er Ke Za Zhi. 2011;13(8):661-4. (article in Chinese)

[308] Jiang ZY, Sun LH, Lin YC, Ma XY, Zheng CT, Zhou GL, Chen F, Zou ST. Effects of dietary glycyl-glutamine on growth performance, small intestinal integrity, and immune responses of weaning piglets challenged with lipopolysaccharide. J Anim Sci. 2009;87(12):4050-6.

[309] Shaw AC, Joshi S, Greenwood H, Panda A, Lord JM. Aging of the innate immune system. Curr Opin Immunol. 2010 Aug;22(4):507-13.

[310] Hummelen R, Vos AP, Land BV, Norren K, Reid G. Altered Host-Microbe Interaction in HIV: A Target for Intervention with Pro- and Prebiotics. Int Rev Immunol. 2010;29(5):485-513.

[311] Klatt NR, Canary LA, Sun X, Vinton CL, Funderburg NT, Morcock DR, Quiñones M, Deming CB, Perkins M, Hazuda DJ, Miller MD, Lederman MM, Segre JA, Lifson JD, Haddad EK, Estes JD, Brenchley JM. Probiotic/prebiotic supplementation of antiretrovirals improves gastrointestinal immunity in SIV-infected macaques. J Clin Invest. 2013 Jan 16. pii: 66227.

[312] Reuter S, Gupta SC, Chaturvedi MM, Aggarwal BB. Oxidative stress, inflammation, and cancer: How are they linked? Free Radic Biol Med. 2010;49(11):1603-16.

[313] http://www.surgeongeneral.gov/library/bonehealth/chapter_4.html#Prevalence

[314] Alarcón T, Gonzalez-Montalvo JI, Gotor P, Madero R, Otero A. A new hierarchical classification for prognosis of hip fracture after 2 years' follow-up. J Nutr Health Aging. 2011;15(10):919-23.

[315] White BL, Fisher WD, Laurin CA. Rate of mortality for elderly patients after fracture of the hip in the 1980's. The Journal of Bone and Joint Surgery. American Volume 1987, 69(9):1335-40.

[316] Chang KP, Center JR, Nguyen TV, Eisman JA. Incidence of hip and other osteoporotic fractures in elderly men and women: Dubbo Osteoporosis Epidemiology Study. J Bone Miner Res. 2004;19(4):532-6.

[317] Delmi M, Rapin CH, Bengoa JM, Bonjour[c] JP, Vasey H, Delmas[d] PD. Dietary supplementation in elderly patients with fractured neck of the femur. Volume 335, Issue 8696, Pages 1013–1016.

[318] JAMA, December 23/30, 1998—Vol 280, No. 24

[319] Nieves JW, Cosman F. Atypical subtrochanteric and femoral shaft fractures and possible association with bisphosphonates. Curr Osteoporos Rep. 2010;8(1):34-9.

[320] Dietary Reference Intakes (DRIs): Recommended Dietary Allowances and Adequate Intakes, Vitamins; Food and Nutrition Board, Institute of Medicine, National Academies

[321] Dietary Reference Intakes (DRIs): Recommended Dietary Allowances and Adequate Intakes, Elements. Food and Nutrition Board, Institute of Medicine, National Academies

[322] Kung AW, Luk KD, Chu LW, Chiu PK. Age-related osteoporosis in Chinese: an evaluation of the response of intestinal calcium absorption and calcitropic hormones to dietary calcium deprivation. Am J Clin Nutr. 1998;68(6):1291-7.

[323] Xu. L. et al, Very low rates of hip fracture in Beijing, People's Republic of China ; The Beijing Osteoprosis Project. Am.J.Epedemiol. 1996; 144 (9): 901-907.

[324] Xia WB, He SL, Xu L, Liu AM, Jiang Y, Li M, Wang O, Xing XP, Sun Y, Cummings SR. Rapidly increasing rates of hip fracture in Beijing, China. J Bone Miner Res. 2011. doi: 10.1002/jbmr.519.

[325] Zalloua PA, Hsu YH, Terwedow H, Zang T, Wu D, Tang G, Li Z, Hong X, Azar ST, Wang B, Bouxsein ML, Brain J, Cummings SR, Rosen CJ, Xu X. Impact of seafood and fruit consumption on bone mineral density. Maturitas. 2007;56(1):1-11.

[326] Tilg H, Moschen AR, Kaser A, Pines A, Dotan I. Gut, inflammation and osteoporosis: basic and clinical concepts. Gut. 2008;57(5):684-94.

[327] Fujita T, Fukase M. Comparison of osteoporosis and calcium intake between Japan and the United States. Proc Soc Exp Biol Med. 1992;200(2):149-52.

[328] http://www.health.harvard.edu/plate/healthy-eating-plate

[329] http://www.choosemyplate.gov/index.html

[330] Bolland MJ, Avenell A, Baron JA, Grey A, MacLennan GS, Gamble GD, Reid IR. Effect of calcium supplements on risk of myocardial infarction and cardiovascular events: meta-analysis. BMJ. 2010; 341:c3691.

[331] Reid IR, Bolland MJ, Sambrook PN, Grey A. Calcium supplementation: balancing the cardiovascular risks. Maturitas. 2011;69(4):289-95.

[332] Nieves JW, Barrett-Connor E, Siris ES, Zion M, Barlas S, Chen YT. Calcium and vitamin D intake influence bone mass, but not short-term fracture risk, in Caucasian postmenopausal women from the National Osteoporosis Risk Assessment (NORA) study. Osteoporos Int. 2008;19(5):673-9.

[333] Feskanich D, Willett WC, Stampfer MJ, Colditz GA. Milk, dietary calcium, and bone fractures in women: a 12-year prospective study. Am J Public Health. 1997;87(6):992-7.

[334] Sharma A, Flom PL, Weedon J, Klein RS. Prospective study of bone mineral density changes in aging men with or at risk for HIV infection. AIDS. 2010;24(15):2337-45. doi:10.1097/QAD.0b013e32833d7da7.

[335] Moskovic DJ, Araujo AB, Lipshultz LI, Khera M. The 20-Year Public Health Impact and Direct Cost of Testosterone Deficiency in U.S. Men. J Sex Med. 2012. doi: 10.1111/j.1743-6109.2012.02944.x.

[336] Strategies for Management of Antiretroviral Therapy (SMART) Study Group, El-Sadr WM, Lundgren J, Neaton JD, Gordin F, Abrams D, Arduino RC, Babiker A, Burman W, Clumeck N et al. CD4+ count-guided interruption of antiretroviral treatment. N Engl J Med. 2006;355(22):2283-96.

[337] Grund B, Peng G, Gibert CL, Hoy JF, Isaksson RL, Shlay JC, Martinez E, Reiss P, Visnegarwala F, Carr AD; INSIGHT SMART Body Composition Substudy Group Continuous antiretroviral therapy decreases bone mineral density. AIDS. 2009;23(12):1519-29.

[338] Hoy J, Grund B, Roediger M, Ensrud KE, Brar I, Colebunders R, De Castro N, Johnson M, Sharma A, Carr A; for the INSIGHT SMART Body Composition Substudy Group Interruption or deferral of antiretroviral therapy reduces markers of bone turnover compared with continuous therapy: The SMART Body Composition substudy. J Bone Miner Res. 2013. doi: 10.1002/jbmr.1861.

[339] Hansen AB, Gerstoft J, Kronborg G, Larsen CS, Pedersen C, Pedersen G, Obel N
Incidence of low and high-energy fractures in persons with and without HIV infection: a Danish population-based cohort study. AIDS. 2012;26(3):285-93.

[340] Yong MK, Elliott JH, Woolley IJ, Hoy JF. Low CD4 count is associated with an increased risk of fragility fracture in HIV-infected patients. J Acquir Immune Defic Syndr. 2011;57(3):205-10.

[341] Martín-Morales R, Ruiz J, Nuño E, Márquez M, Santos J, Palacios R. Bone turnover markers in HIV-infected patients before starting antiretroviral therapy. J Int AIDS Soc. 2012 Nov 11;15(6):18321.

[342] Cervero M, Agud J, Torres R, Jusdado J. Vitamin D status in an urban Spanish HIV-infected patient cohort and its relationship with most frequent antiretroviral therapy regimens. J Int AIDS Soc. 2012;15(6):18323.

[343] Xu R. Effect of whey protein on the proliferation and differentiation of osteoblasts. J Dairy Sci. 2009;92(7):3014-8.

[344] Tsuji-Naito K, Jack RW. Concentrated bovine milk whey active proteins facilitate osteogenesis through activation of the JNK-ATF4 pathway. Biosci Biotechnol Biochem. 2012;76(6):1150-4.

[345] Bech A, Van Bentum P, Telting D, Gisolf J et al. Treatment of calcium and vitamin D deficiency in HIV-positive men on tenofovir-containing antiretroviral therapy. HIV Clin Trials. 2012;13(6):350-6.

[346] I have no ties to this company.

[347] Ribeiro RT, Afonso RA, Guarino MP, Macedo MP. Loss of postprandial insulin sensitization during aging. J Gerontol A Biol Sci Med Sci. 2008;63(6):560-5.

[348] Tilg H, Moschen AR. Inflammatory mechanisms in the regulation of insulin resistance. Mol Med. 2008;14(3-4):222-31.

[349] Orchard TJ, Temprosa M, Barrett-Connor E, Fowler S, Goldberg R, Mather K, Marcovina S, Montez M, Ratner R, Saudek C, Sherif H, Watson K; The Diabetes Prevention Program Outcomes Study Research Group; prepared on behalf of the DPPOS Research Group Long-term effects of the Diabetes Prevention Program interventions on cardiovascular risk factors: a report from the DPP Outcomes Study. Diabet Med. 2013; 30(1): 46-55.

[350] Liese AD, Weis KE, Schulz M, Tooze JA. Food intake patterns associated with incident type 2 diabetes: the Insulin Resistance Atherosclerosis Study. Diabetes Care. 2009;32(2):263-8.

351 Lim S, Won H, Kim Y, Jang M, Jyothi KR, Kim Y, Dandona P et al. Antioxidant enzymes induced by repeated intake of excess energy in the form of high-fat, high-carbohydrate meals are not sufficient to block oxidative stress in healthy lean individuals. Br J Nutr. 2011;106(10):1544-51.

352 Abete I, Goyenechea E, Zulet MA, Martínez JA. Obesity and metabolic syndrome: potential benefit from specific nutritional components. Nutr Metab Cardiovasc Dis. 2011;21 Suppl 2:B1-15.

353 Tappy L, Lê KA, Tran C, Paquot N. Fructose and metabolic diseases: new findings, new questions. Nutrition 2010;26(11-12):1044-9.

354 Rayssiguier Y, Gueux E, Nowacki W, Rock E, Mazur A. High fructose consumption combined with low dietary magnesium intake may increase the incidence of the metabolic syndrome by inducing inflammation. Magnes Res. 2006; 19(4):237-43.

355 Rosanoff A. Rising Ca:Mg intake ratio from food in USA Adults: a concern? Magnes Res. 2010;23(4):S181-93.

356 Barbagallo M, Belvedere M, Dominguez LJ. Magnesium homeostasis and aging. Magnes Res. 2009;22(4):235-46.

357 Williams AD, Almond J, Ahuja KD, Beard DC et al. Cardiovascular and metabolic effects of community based resistance training in an older population. J Sci Med Sport. 2011;14(4):331-7.

358 Tomlinson JW, Finney J, Gay C, Hughes BA, Hughes SV, Stewart PM. Impaired glucose tolerance and insulin resistance are associated with increased adipose 11beta-hydroxysteroid dehydrogenase type 1 expression and elevated hepatic 5alpha-reductase activity. Diabetes. 2008;57(10):2652-60.

359 Shearer GC, Savinova OV, Harris WS. Fish Oil –How doies it reduce plasma triglycerides? Biochem Biophys Acta. 2012; 1921(5):843-51.

360 Ruggenenti P, Cattaneo D, Loriga G, Ledda F, Motterlini N, Gherardi G, Orisio S, Remuzzi G. Ameliorating hypertension and insulin resistance in subjects at increased cardiovascular risk: effects of acetyl-L-carnitine therapy. Hypertension. 2009;54(3):567-74.

361 Bugianesi E, Moscatiello S, Ciaravella MF, Marchesini G. Insulin resistance in nonalcoholic fatty liver disease. Curr Pharm Des. 2010 ;16(17):1941-51.

362 Ziyadeh N, McAfee AT, Koro C, Landon J, Arnold Chan K. The thiazolidinediones rosiglitazone and pioglitazone and the risk of coronary heart disease: a retrospective cohort study using a US health insurance database. Clin Ther. 2009;31(11):2665-77.

363 Mamtani R, Haynes K, Bilker WB, Vaughn DJ, Strom BL, Glanz K, Lewis JD. Association Between Longer Therapy With Thiazolidinediones and Risk of Bladder Cancer: A Cohort Study. J Natl Cancer Inst. 2012; 104(18):1411-21.

364 http://lpi.oregonstate.edu/infocenter/othernuts/carnitine/

365 von Hurst PR, Stonehouse W, Coad J. Vitamin D supplementation reduces insulin resistance in South Asian women living in New Zealand who are insulin resistant and vitamin D deficient - a randomised, placebo-controlled trial. Br J Nutr. 2010;103(4):549-55.

366 Wang ZQ, Cefalu WT. Current concepts about chromium supplementation in type 2 diabetes and insulin resistance. Curr Diab Rep. 2010;10(2):145-51.

367 Clandinin MT, Cheema S, Field CJ, Baracos VE. Dietary lipids influence insulin action. Ann N Y Acad Sci. 1993;683:151-63.

368 Wilmore DW. The effect of glutamine supplementation in patients following elective surgery and accidental injury. J Nutr. 2001;131(9 Suppl):2543S-9S; discussion 2550S-1S

369 Samocha-Bonet D, Wong O, Synnott EL, Piyaratna N, Douglas A, Gribble FM, Holst JJ, Chisholm DJ, Greenfield JR. Glutamine reduces postprandial glycemia and augments the glucagon-like peptide-1 response in type 2 diabetes patients. J Nutr. 2011;141(7):1233-8.

370 Menge BA, Schrader H, Ritter PR, Ellrichmann M, Uhl W, Schmidt WE, Meier JJ. Selective amino acid deficiency in patients with impaired glucose tolerance and type 2 diabetes. Regul Pept. 2010;160(1-3):75-80.

371 Krause MS, McClenaghan NH, Flatt PR, de Bittencourt PI, Murphy C, Newsholme P. L-arginine is essential for pancreatic β-cell functional integrity, metabolism and defense from inflammatory challenge. J Endocrinol. 2011;211(1):87-97.

372 Silva N, Atlantis E, Ismail K. A review of the association between depression and insulin resistance: pitfalls of secondary analyses or a promising new approach to prevention of type 2 diabetes? Curr Psychiatry Rep. 2012;14(1):8-14.

373 Stuart MJ, Baune BT. Depression and type 2 diabetes: inflammatory mechanisms of a psychoneuroendocrine co-morbidity. Neurosci Biobehav Rev. 2012;36(1):658-76.

374 Ajilore O, Haroon E, Kumaran S, Darwin C, Binesh N, Mintz J, Miller J, Thomas MA, Kumar A. Measurement of brain metabolites in patients with type 2 diabetes and major depression using proton magnetic resonance spectroscopy. Neuropsychopharmacology. 2007;32(6):1224-31.

375 Young LS, Bye R, Scheltinga M, Ziegler TR, Jacobs DO, Wilmore DW. Patients receiving glutamine-supplemented intravenous feedings report an improvement in mood. JPEN J Parenter Enteral Nutr. 1993;17(5):422-7.

376 Maggio M, Lauretani F, Ceda GP, Bandinelli S, Basaria S, Ble A, Egan J, Paolisso G, Najjar S, Jeffrey Metter E, Valenti G, Guralnik JM, Ferrucci L. Association between hormones and metabolic syndrome in older Italian men. J Am Geriatr Soc. 2006;54(12):1832-8.

377 Kintzel PE, Chase SL, Schultz LM, O'Rourke TJ. Increased risk of metabolic syndrome, diabetes mellitus, and cardiovascular disease in men receiving androgen deprivation therapy for prostate cancer. Pharmacotherapy. 2008;28(12):1511-22.

378 Atlantis E, Lange K, Martin S, Haren MT, Taylor A, O'Loughlin PD, Marshall V, Wittert GA. Testosterone and modifiable risk factors associated with diabetes in men. Maturitas. 2011;68(3):279-85.

379 Reynolds AC, Dorrian J, Liu PY, Van Dongen HP, Wittert GA, Harmer LJ, Banks S. Impact of five nights of sleep restriction on glucose metabolism, leptin and testosterone in young adult men. PLoS One. 2012;7(7):e41218.

380 Hadigan C, Corcoran C, Stanley T, Piecuch S, Klibanski A, Grinspoon S. Fasting hyperinsulinemia in human immunodeficiency virus-infected men: relationship to body composition, gonadal function, and protease inhibitor use. J Clin Endocrinol Metab. 2000;85(1):35-41.

381 Morgentaler A. Testosterone therapy in men with prostate cancer: scientific and ethical considerations. J Urol. 2013;189(1 Suppl):S26-33.

[382] Yasui T, Matsui S, Tani A, Kunimi K, Yamamoto S, Irahara M. Androgen in postmenopausal women. J Med Invest. 2012;59(1-2):12-27.

[383] Villareal DT, Holloszy JO. Effect of DHEA on abdominal fat and insulin action in elderly women and men: a randomized controlled trial. JAMA. 2004;292(18):2243-8.

[384] Nair KS, Rizza RA, O'Brien P, Dhatariya K, Short KR, Nehra A, Vittone JL, Klee GG, Basu A, Basu R, Cobelli C, Toffolo G, Dalla Man C, Tindall DJ, Melton LJ 3rd, Smith GE, Khosla S, Jensen MD. DHEA in elderly women and DHEA or testosterone in elderly men. N Engl J Med. 2006;355(16):1647-59.

[385] Lee NK, Sowa H, Hinoi E, Ferron M, Ahn JD, Confavreux C, Dacquin R, Mee PJ, McKee MD, Jung DY, Zhang Z, Kim JK, Mauvais-Jarvis F, Ducy P, Karsenty G. Endocrine regulation of energy metabolism by the skeleton. Cell. 2007 Aug 10;130(3):456-69.

[386] Park K, Steffes M, Lee DH, Himes JH, Jacobs DR Jr. Association of inflammation with worsening HOMA-insulin resistance. Diabetologia. 2009;52(11):2337-44.

[387] Ylönen K, Alfthan G, Groop L, Saloranta C, Aro A, Virtanen SM. Dietary intakes and plasma concentrations of carotenoids and tocopherols in relation to glucose metabolism in subjects at high risk of type 2 diabetes: the Botnia Dietary Study. Am J Clin Nutr. 2003 ;77(6):1434-41.

[388] Fang F, Kang Z, Wong C. Vitamin E tocotrienols improve insulin sensitivity through activating peroxisome proliferator-activated receptors. Mol Nutr Food Res. 2010;54(3):345-52.

[389] Paolisso G, Balbi V, Volpe C, Varricchio G, Gambardella A, Saccomanno F, Ammendola S, Varricchio M, D'Onofrio F. Metabolic benefits deriving from chronic vitamin C supplementation in aged non-insulin dependent diabetics. J Am Coll Nutr. 1995;14(4):387-92.

[390] Rizzo MR, Abbatecola AM, Barbieri M, Vietri MT, Cioffi M, Grella R, Molinari A, Forsey R, Powell J, Paolisso G. Evidence for anti-inflammatory effects of combined administration of vitamin E and C in older persons with impaired fasting glucose: impact on insulin action. J Am Coll Nutr. 2008;27(4):505-11.

[391] Lautt WW, Ming Z, Legare DJ. Attenuation of age- and sucrose-induced insulin resistance and syndrome X by a synergistic antioxidant cocktail: the AMIS syndrome and HISS hypothesis. Can J Physiol Pharmacol. 2010;88(3):313-23.

[392] Lautt WW, Macedo MP, Sadri P, Takayama S, Duarte Ramos F, Legare DJ. Hepatic parasympathetic (HISS) control of insulin sensitivity determined by feeding and fasting. Am J Physiol Gastrointest Liver Physiol. 2001;281(1):G29-36.

[393] Mietus-Snyder ML, Shigenaga MK, Suh JH, Shenvi SV, Lal A, McHugh T, Olson D, Lilienstein J, Krauss RM, Gildengoren G, McCann JC, Ames BN. A nutrient-dense, high-fiber, fruit-based supplement bar increases HDL cholesterol, particularly large HDL, lowers homocysteine, and raises glutathione in a 2-wk trial. FASEB J. 2012;26(8):3515-27.

[394] Ringseis R, Keller J, Eder K. Role of carnitine in the regulation of glucose homeostasis and insulin sensitivity: evidence from in vivo and in vitro studies with carnitine supplementation and carnitine deficiency. Eur J Nutr. 2012;51(1):1-18.

[395] Golbidi S, Badran M, Laher I. Diabetes and alpha lipoic Acid. Front Pharmacol. 2011;2:69.

[396] Padmalayam I. Targeting mitochondrial oxidative stress through lipoic Acid synthase: a novel strategy to manage diabetic cardiovascular disease. Cardiovasc Hematol Agents Med Chem. 2012;10(3):223-33.

[397] Watts GF, Playford DA, Croft KD, Ward NC, Mori TA, Burke V. Coenzyme Q(10) improves endothelial dysfunction of the brachial artery in Type II diabetes mellitus. Diabetologia. 2002;45(3):420-6.

[398] Hamilton SJ, Chew GT, Watts GF. Coenzyme Q10 improves endothelial dysfunction in statin-treated type 2 diabetic patients. Diabetes Care. 2009;32(5):810-2.

[399] Gelato MC, Mynarcik DC, Quick JL, Steigbigel RT, Fuhrer J, Brathwaite CE, Brebbia JS, Wax MR, McNurlan MA. Improved insulin sensitivity and body fat distribution in HIV-infected patients treated with rosiglitazone: a pilot study. J Acquir Immune Defic Syndr 2002;31(2):163-70.

[400] Abete I, Goyenechea E, Zulet MA, Martínez JA. Obesity and metabolic syndrome: potential benefit from specific nutritional components. Nutr Metab Cardiovasc Dis. 2011;21 Suppl 2:B1-15.

[401] Kim DJ, Xun P, Liu K, Loria C, Yokota K, Jacobs DR Jr, He K. Magnesium intake in relation to systemic inflammation, insulin resistance, and the incidence of diabetes. Diabetes Care. 2010;33(12):2604-10.

[402] Das UN. A defect in the activity of Delta6 and Delta5 desaturases may be a factor in the initiation and progression of atherosclerosis. Prostaglandins Leukot Essent Fatty Acids. 200;76(5):251-68.

[403] Horrobin DF. Essential fatty acids in the management of impaired nerve function in diabetes. Diabetes. 1997;46 Suppl 2:S90-3.

[404] Han T, Bai JF, Liu W, Hu YM. A systemic review and Meta-analysis of α-lipoic acid in the treatment of diabetic peripheral neuropathy. Eur J Endocrinol. 2012 Jul 25. [Epub ahead of print]

[405] Stracke H, Lindemann A, Federlin K. A benfotiamine-vitamin B combination in treatment of diabetic polyneuropathy. Exp Clin Endocrinol Diabetes. 1996;104(4):311-6.

[406] Zhang W, Cox AG, Taylor EW. Hepatitis C virus encodes a selenium-dependent glutathione peroxidase gene. Implications for oxidative stress as a risk factor in progression to hepatocellular carcinoma. Med Klin (Munich). 1999;94 Suppl 3:2-6.

[407] Lu SC. Regulation of hepatic glutathione synthesis: current concepts and controversies. FASEB J; 13(10):1169-83.

[408] Marmor M, Alcabes P, Titus S, Frenkel K, Krasinski K, Penn A, Pero RW. Low serum thiol levels predict shorter times-to-death among HIV-infected injecting drug users.AIDS. 1997;11(11):1389-93.

[409] R Buhl. Imbalance between oxidants and antioxidants in the lungs of HIV-seropositive individuals. Chemico-Biological Interactions 1994, 91:147-158.

[410] Rosser BG Gores GJ. Liver cell necrosis: cellular mechanisms and clinical implications. Gastroenterology. 1995;108(1):252-75. Review.

[411] Look MP, Rockstroh JK, Rao GS, Kreuzer K_A, Barton S, Lemoch H, Sudhop T, Hoch J, Stockinger K, Spengler U, Sauerbruch T. Serum selenium, plasma glutathione (GSH) and erythrocyte glutathione peroxidase (GSH-Px)-levels in asymptomatic versus symptomatic human immunodeficiency virus-1 (HIV-1)-infection. Euro J Clin Nutr 1997 51:266-72.

[412] Sulkowski MS, Thomas DL, Chaisson Re, Moore RD. Hepatotoxicity associated with antiretroviral therapy in adults infected with Human Immunodeficiency virus and the role of hepatitis C or B virus infection. JAMA 2000; 283(1)74-80.

413 Walmsley SL, Winn LM, Harrison ML, Uetrecht JP, Wells PG. Oxidative stress and thiol depletion in plasma and peripheral blood lymphocytes from HIV-infected patients: toxicological and pathological implications. AIDS 1997;11:1689-97.

414 Peterson JD, Herzenberg LA, Vasquez K, Waltenbaugh C. Glutathione levels in antigen-presenting cells modulate Th1 versus Th2 response patterns. Proc Natl Acad Sci U S A. 1998;95(6):3071-6.

415 Aukrust P, Svardal AM, Muller F, Lunden B, Nordoy I, Froland SS. Markedly disturbed glutathione redox status in CD45RA+CD4+ lymphocytes in human immunodeficiency virus Type 1 infection is associated with selective depletion of this lymphocyte subset. Blood 1996; 88(7):2626-2633.

416 Weiss L, Hildt E, Hofschneider PH. Anti-hepatitis B virus activity of N-acetyl-L-cysteine (NAC): new aspects of a well-established drug. 1996 Antiviral Res 32(1):43-53.

417 Beloqui O, Prieto J, Suarez M et al. N-acetyl cysteine enhances the response to interferon-alpha in chronic hepatitis C: a pilot study. J Interferon Res 1993;13(4):279-82.

418 Diaz PT, King MA, Pacht ER, et al. Increased susceptibility to pulmonary emphysema among HIV-seropositive smokers. Ann Intern Med 2000; 132:369-372.

419 Herzenberg LA, De Rosa SC, Dubs JG, Roederer M, Anderson MT, Ela SW, Deresinski SC, Herzenberg LA. Glutathione deficiency is associated with impaired survival in HIV disease.Proc Natl Acad Sci U S A. 1997;94(5):1967-72.

420 Mynarcik DC, McNurlan MA, Steigbigel RT, Fuhrer J, Gelato MC. Association of severe insulin resistance with both loss of limb fat and elevated serum tumor necrosis factor receptor levels in HIV lipodystrophy. J Acquir Immune Defic Syndr. 2000;25(4):312-21

421 Christeff, Melchior Increased serum interferon alpha in HIV-1 associated lipodystrophy syndrome. Eur J Clin Investig. 2002; 32(1):43-50.

422 Shevitz A, Wanke CA, Falutz J, Kotler D. Clinical perspectives on HIV-associated lipodystrophy syndrome: an update. AIDS 2001; 15:1917-30.

423 Walker KZ, O'Dea K, Nicholson GC. Dietary composition affects regional body fat distribution and levels of dehydroepiandrosterone sulphate (DHEAS) in post-menopausal women with Type 2 diabetes. Eur J Clin Nutr 1999 53(9):700-5.

424 Dalakas C, Illa I, Pezeshkpour GH et al. Mitochondrial myopathy caused by long-term zidovudine therapy. Ne Engl J Med 1990 322:1098-1105.

425 Lewis W, Dalakas M.. Mitochondrial toxicity of antiviral drugs. Nature Medicine 1995 1(5):417-22..

426 Valantin MA, Bittar R, de Truchis P, Bollens D, Slama L, Giral P, Bonnefont-Rousselot D, Pétour P, Aubron-Olivier C, Costagliola D, Katlama C; TOTEM trial group Switching the nucleoside reverse transcriptase inhibitor backbone to tenofovir disoproxil fumarate + emtricitabine promptly improves triglycerides and low-density lipoprotein cholesterol in dyslipidaemic patients. J Antimicrob Chemother. 2010;65(3):556-61.

427 Abraham P, Ramamoorthy H, Isaac B. Depletion of the cellular antioxidant system contributes to tenofovir disoproxil fumarate - induced mitochondrial damage and increased oxido-nitrosative stress in the kidney. J Biomed Sci. 2013;20:61.

428 Meininger G, Hadigan C, Laposata M, Brown J, Rabe J, Louca J, Aliabadi N, Grinspoon S. Elevated concentrations of free fatty acids are associated with increased insulin response to standard glucose challenge in human immunodeficiency virus-infected subjects with fat redistribution. Metabolism. 2002;51(2):260-6.

429 Roden M, Price TB, Perseghin G, Petersen KF, Rothman DL, Cline GW, Shulman GI. Mechanism of free fatty acid-induced insulin resistance in humans. 1996; 97:2859-2865.

430 Hadigan C, Corcoran C, Stanley T, Piecuch S, Klibanski A, Grinspoon S. Fasting hyperinsulinemia in human immunodeficiency virus-infected men: relationship to body composition, gonadal function, and protease inhibitor use. J Clin Endocrinol Metab. 2000;85(1):35-41.

431 de la Asuncion JG, del Olmo ML, Sastre J et al. AZT treatment induces molecular and ultrastructural oxidative damage to muscle mitochondria. Prevention by antioxidant vitamins. J Clin Invest 1998; 102(1):4-9.

432 Mingrone G, Rosa G, Di Rocco P, Manco M, Capristo E, Castagneto M, Vettor R, Gasbarrini G, Greco AV. Skeletal muscle triglycerides lowering is associated with net improvement of insulin sensitivity, TNF-a reduction and GLUT4 expression enhancement. Int J Obesity 2002, 26:1165-1172.

433 Roubenoff R, Schmitz H, Bairos L, Layne J, Potts E, Cloutier GJ, Denry F.
Reduction of abdominal obesity in lipodystrophy associated with human immunodeficiency virus infection by means of diet and exercise: case report and proof of principle. Clin Infect Dis 2002 Feb 1;34(3):390-3.

434 Urberg M, Zemel MB. Evidence for synergism between chromium and nicotinic acid in the control of glucose tolerance in elderly humans. Metabolism. 1987;36(9):896-9.

435 Meininger G, Hadigan C, Laposata M, Brown J, Rabe J, Louca J, Aliabadi N, Grinspoon S. Elevated concentrations of free fatty acids are associated with increased insulin response to standard glucose challenge in human immunodeficiency virus-infected subjects with fat redistribution. Metabolism. 2002;51(2):260-6.

436 Hadigan C, Rabe J, Meininger G, Aliabadi N, Breu J, Grinspoon S. Inhibition of lipolysis improves insulin sensitivity in protease inhibitor-treated HIV-infected men with fat redistribution. Am J Clin Nutr. 2003;77(2):490-4.

437 Hadigan C, Jeste S, Anderson EJ, Tsay R, Cyr H, Grinspoon S. Modifiable dietary habits and their relation to metabolic abnormalities in men and women with human immunodeficiency virus infection and fat redistribution. Clin Infect Dis. 2001;33(5):710-7.

438 Grimaldi PA, Teboul L, Inadera H, Gaillard D, Amri EZ. Trans-differentiation of myoblasts to adipoblasts: triggering effects of fatty acids and thiazolidinediones. Prostaglandins, Leukotrienes and Essentail Fatty Acids 1997 57(1):71-75.

439 Gelato MC, Mynarcik DC, Quick JL, Steigbigel RT, Fuhrer J, Brathwaite CE, Brebbia JS, Wax MR, McNurlan MA. Improved insulin sensitivity and body fat distribution in HIV-infected patients treated with rosiglitazone: a pilot study. J Acquir Immune Defic Syndr. 2002;31(2):163-70.

440 Schoonjans K, Staels B, Auwerx J. Role of the peroxisome proliferator-activated receptor (PPAR) in mediating the effects of fibrates and fatty acids on gene expression. J Lipid Res 37(5):907-25.

[441] Thoennes SR, Tate PL, Price TM, Kilgore MW. Differential transcriptional activation of peroxisome proliferators-activated receptor gamma by omega-3 and omega-6 fatty acids in MCF-7 cells. Mol Cell Endocrinol 2000; 160 (1-2):67-73.

[442] Yarasheski KE, Tebas P, Claxton S, Marin D, Coleman T, Powderly WG, Semenkovich CF. Visceral adiposity, C-peptide levels, and low lipase activities predict HIV-dyslipidemia. Am J Physiol Endocrinol Metab. 2003;285(4):E899-905.

[443] Connor WE, DeFrancesco CA, Connor SL. N-3 fatty acids from fish oil. Effects on plasma lipoproteins and hypertriglyceridemic patients. Ann N Y Acad Sci 1993; 683:16-34.

[444] Moretti S, Famularo G, Marcellini S, Boschini A, Santini G, Trinchieri V, Lucci L, Alesse E, De Simone C. L-carnitine reduces lymphocyte apoptosis and oxidant stress in HIV-1-infected subjects treated with zidovudine and didanosine. Antioxid Redox Signal. 2002;4(3):391-403.

[445] Fliers E et al. HIV-associated adipose redistribution syndrome as a selective autonomic neuropathy. The Lancet 362: 1758 – 1760, 2003.

[446] Baldewicz T, Goodkin K, Feaster DJ, Blaney NT, Kumar M, Kumar A, Shor-Posner G, Baum M. Plasma pyridoxine deficiency is related to increased psychological distress in recently bereaved homosexual men. Psychosom Med. 1998;60(3):297-308.

[447] Baldewicz TT, Goodkin K, Blaney NT, Shor-Posner G, Kumar M, Wilkie FL, Baum MK, Eisdorfer C. Cobalamin level is related to self-reported and clinically rated mood and to syndromal depression in bereaved HIV-1(+) and HIV-1(-) homosexual men. J Psychosom Res. 2000;48(2):177-85.

[448] Murasato Y, Harada Y, Ikeda M, Nakashima Y, Hayashida Y. Effect of magnesium deficiency on autonomic circulatory regulation in conscious rats. Hypertension. 1999;34(2):247-52.

[449] Xu M, Dai W, Deng X. Effects of magnesium sulfate on brain mitochondrial respiratory function in rats after experimental traumatic brain injury. Chin J Traumatol. 2002 Dec;5(6):361-4.

[450] Watanabe T, Kaji R, Oka N, Bara W, Kimura J. Ultra-high dose methylcobalamin promotes nerve regeneration in experimental acrylamide neuropathy. J Neurol Sci. 1994;122(2):140-3.

[451] Bernstein AL, Dinesen JS. Brief communication: effect of pharmacologic doses of vitamin B6 on carpal tunnel syndrome, electroencephalographic results, and pain. J Am Coll Nutr. 1993;12(1):73-6.

[452] Ruhnau KJ, Meissner HP, Finn JR, Reljanovic M, Lobisch M, Schütte K, Nehrdich D, Tritschler HJ, Mehnert H, Ziegler D. Effects of 3-week oral treatment with the antioxidant thioctic acid (alpha-lipoic acid) in symptomatic diabetic polyneuropathy. Diabet Med. 1999;16(12):1040-3.

[453] William Daley, MD; How Tong Ren Works, at www tomtam com

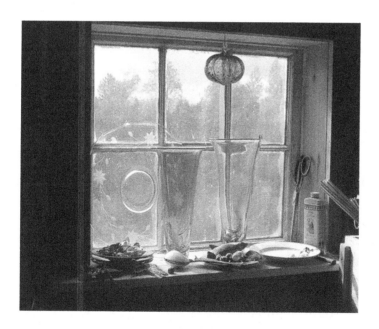

[454] http://www.flickr.com/photos/43071680@N00/ Thanks to Karen Larsen for the delicious photos used throughout the book.

As of Winter, 2014, a simple but comprehensive supplement plan to both nurture immune cells and support ant-inflammatory enzymes in the body looks like the list of items seen below.

(There are still more items to use to fix metabolism, and those are reviewed throughout the book. This list is a basic support plan.
It could cost about $1.00 a day with careful shopping.)

Hierarchy of Supplement Intervention

1. **Enhanced Multivitamin**: 100% RDA for usual vitamins, 100 mg Magnesium, 100 mcg Selenium, plus10 X RDA B-complex, vit C & E.

Pick one:

50+ Men by Supernutrition,	NYBC	$20/mo
50+ Women by Supernutrition	NYBC	$20/mo
Active Senior Multivitamins by Rainbow Light	Vitamin Shoppe	$9/mo
Two Per Day Tablets* by Life Extension	Vitamin Shoppe	$8.50/mo
Active 50+ Once Daily Multivitamin & Minerals	Trader Joe's	$6/mo

NYBC = newyorkbuyersclub.org (also available at Whole Foods Markets)

2. **Glutathione support**
   Improve CD4 count, lower LFT's in HCV, boost energy/Lean Body Mass

   L-glutamine- 5 grams (1heaping teaspoon powder) The Vitamin Shoppe or NYBC

3. **Mitochondrial support and Natural Killer cell fuel**.
   Antioxidant, and helps reverse neuropathy and fatigue

Co-enzyme Q10 100 mg, 1/day   NYBC, Trader Joe's, Vit. Shoppe

4. **Probiotics: JarroDophilus eps**, 1/day …   NYBC, Vitamin Shoppe
prevents leaky gut, lowers cholesterol, lowers inflammation in liver.

Depending on the amount of fish, seeds and nuts you eat each day, you may add:

5. **Essential Fatty Acids** & phospholipids .   NYBC, Vit Shoppe or Trader Joes
Maintain arterial health, & peripheral lipase and nitric oxide functions.

Omega 3 EPA/DHA fatty acids: > 800 mg/day as 1-2 gms **Fish Oils**

Omega 6 GLA **Evening Primrose Oil**: 1000 – 1300 mg pill, take 1-2 per day
   This fixes dry skin caused by proteases and raises good HDL cholesterol.

Made in the USA
Monee, IL
31 March 2024

56086597R00090